THE TREATMENT OF PTSD COMORBID CONDITION

INCLUDING: ADDICTION; CHRONIC PAIN; COMPLEX PTSD; DEMENTIA; DEPRESSION; SLEEP DISORDER; SURVIVOR'S GUILT; TRAUMATIC BRAIN INJURY.

George L. Lindenfeld, Ph.D.
Diplomate in Clinical Psychology

"When you're born, a light is switched on, a light which shines up through your life.

As you get older the light still reaches you, sparkling as it comes up through your memories. And if you're lucky as you travel forward through time, you'll bring the whole of yourself along with you, gathering your skirts and leaving nothing behind, nothing to obscure the light.

But if a Bad Thing happens, part of you is seared into place, and trapped for ever at that time. The rest of you moves onward, dealing with all the todays and tomorrows, but something, some part of you, is left behind.

That part blocks the light, colours the rest of your life, but worse than that, it's alive. Trapped for ever at that moment, and alone in the dark, that part of you is still alive."

Michael Marshall Smith, Only Forward

Contents:

Praise:

For the practitioner interested in assisting those with PTSD, this book is a must-read. I had the privilege of recently meeting with Dr. George Lindenfeld and putting my skepticism about this new method directly to the test - by requesting a session to address an unresolved stuck trauma. Just imaging it would make my insides cringe, my fingers wrap into a tight ball, and I would exert all of my effort in trying to push it out of my mind.

Although I am a practitioner of EMDR, and of Neurofeedback as well, these interventions were unsuccessful in making headway with this particular disturbing memory. When Dr. Lindenfeld tuned into the resonant frequency of the target, it was like an accelerator being pushed down on a motorcycle zooming out from 0 – 60 mph in one second.

The target lit up like a ball of fire, and my sympathetic nervous system engaged (huffing and puffing for breath, heart racing, sweating, cringing/squirming, tensing and bracing my muscles. While this was happening, a curious visualization came to my mind involving a mending of my trauma. My breathing slowed, and in what seemed like only moments later, Dr. Lindenfeld stopped the sound.

The result, after only 5 minutes of the binaural beat, was at least a 50% decrease in the intensity of the trauma. If I visualize it now, I no longer cringe or try to push it out of my mind. It goes away on its own in a moment. This was no placebo, and this did not happen with any other method.

I slept well through half the night, and had a weird dream during the second half. By the next day, the improvement level had remained at least 50% improved. Absolutely remarkable! I have noticed other positive improvements such as less anxiety and tension when I drive a car.

I beckon all mental health professionals working with psychological trauma in its many forms to 'take the skeptic test' and undergo a short session of RESET Therapy with a clinician who has been properly trained and certified in its use. If your experience is anything like mine, you will feel a burst of excitement, want to seek more training, get the word out to colleagues, and realize that careful research needs be conducted by those of us who seek to remediate trauma.

Dr. Lindenfeld is to be commended for developing the RESET Therapy protocol, a truly revolutionary, brief, minimally invasive, and effective treatment for PTSD and related conditions. A masterful clinician and teacher, he is a humane, compassionate individual who at age 77 (when others are retired) has dedicated his life to training and certifying others in the RESET Therapy method, promulgating research studies and information about the method, and committing himself to the goal of reducing the suffering experienced by persons exposed to trauma, especially Veterans. Dr. Lindenfeld, thank you for a truly wonderful and lasting gift!

Dr. John Hummer - Licensed Clinical Psychologist

Who is this book for?

In my first book, *Ending the Nightmare of PTSD*, I choose to focus on our combat Veterans and their significant others, in order to instill a seed of hope where before, there has been prevailing despair. My intent was to inform our service men and women as well as their loved ones that there now exists a rapid and noninvasive way to end the daily suffering incurred as a result of their combat related sacrifices. I choose to do this to replace the pervasive and erroneous belief that too many of our mental health professionals have about PTSD being a lifelong psychic injury that cannot be healed.

My second book: (*Brain On Fire: A Therapist's Guide to Extinguishing the Flames of PTSD*), was designed for those healers who seek an alternative, revolutionary approach based on a hypothesis that although PTSD is triggered by trauma, it is really a disease of memory.

I challenged healers to question status quo beliefs about the permanency of PTSD and to join me in an exciting new adventure into a world of transformative opportunity by understanding and then implementing a treatment I have come to call RESET Therapy (Reconsolidation Enhancement through Stimulation of Emotional Triggers).

This third book in the series (*The Treatment of PTSD Comorbid Conditions: Including: Addiction; Chronic Pain; Complex PTSD; Dementia; Depression; Sleep Disorder; Survivor's Guilt; Traumatic Brain Disorder* has been created for the purpose of detailing how varied circuits involved in the above conditions may be remediated. The term comorbid generally refers to at least two different disorders that simultaneously occur in the same person. Thus, each chapter is focused upon a specific comorbid condition that frequently accompanies PTSD.

My perspective is that generally, each of these conditions represents a facet of the PTSD neuronal network in the brain. I believe that we can refer to it as a multi-faceted diamond although what is reflected from this undesirable gem is black light. I have found that at times, when the core trauma circuit is reset, the other conditions may normalize as well.

On other occasions, a specific facet of the circuit requires an individualized 'tuning in' so that the binaural sound resonates with that specific target. Furthermore, conditions such as depression are amenable to this type of treatment in their own right, independent of the presence or absence of trauma. Thus, the practitioner can apply RESET Therapy within the context of multiple and varied clinical situations.

My review of current PTSD literature suggests that presently a micro focus dominates research efforts absent of an overview systemic perspective of the condition. I found one recent book (2016) that diverges from this ever-narrowing perspective taking a much broader and comprehensive view. The authors report that:

"Post-traumatic stress disorder (PTSD) has a prevalence of 6.8% among the American population and an even greater prevalence among combat veterans. The conventional view of PTSD has been to view it as a psychological adjustment disorder characterized by depression and anxiety in response to stressful circumstances. Recently, however, it has become apparent that it is much more than a psychological adjustment disorder.

This began with the appreciation of the fact that dementia is much more common in PTSD than earlier thought, suggesting neurological changes associated with the disorder. There is now evidence for psychiatric changes (e.g., mood disorders, substance use and abuse), cardiovascular changes, auto-immune changes (e.g., rheumatoid arthritis), tumorigenic changes, etc. (Bukhbinder & Schulz, 2016)."

I included the above material because it is my belief that the authors of this book are on the right track. My own perspective is that human beings have not yet adapted to a level necessary for them to sustain the pressures and stresses of modern life. Rather, when we experience trauma, our minds are programmed at a genetic level to go into a defensive, protective mode to ensure our survival.

Understanding this self-protective cortical mechanism permits us to turn the growth switch back on by resetting the altered and frozen neuronal circuitry. Each chapter of this text addresses different comorbid features that are frequently associated with PTSD. Case studies will be provided where possible to illustrate the potential for change that RESET Therapy can offer.

Originally, I thought that seven chapters would suffice however, I was stunned by the concurrence and elevated percentages of sleep disorders in those with chronic PTSD. Amazingly, this was the case even in those Veterans who were alleged to have 'successfully' completed treatment for PTSD. How can we be so blind?

I've come to the conclusion that unless the comorbid condition of sleep disorder is eliminated through the specified 'gold standard' or experimental treatment, the PTSD neuronal network remains activated even if this is at a subconscious level. To state it differently, if the sleep disturbance isn't normalized, I consider the treatment to be a failure in re-establishing a homeostatic systemic balance in the afflicted individual. Although this has not yet been proven, the hypothesis becomes readably testable. I will plan to explore this thesis in the near future.

Once again, I need to state that this is not a DIY (Do It Yourself) project. Beyond what you have read in my earlier books or what you are to read in this book, you will need to implement specialized 'hands on' training leading to your being certified in RESET Therapy before applying this treatment in clinical settings.

Foreword

It is a pleasure and a privilege to write the foreword to Dr. George Lindenfeld's latest book describing his use of neuromodulated sound on conditions that have been found to co-occur with PTSD. Indeed, Dr. Lindenfeld has concentrated his attention on post-traumatic stress disorder (PTSD) which has recently come into public and media prominence due to its high prevalence in military Veterans.

Dr. Lindenfeld has also included in "Chapter Two: Traumatic Brain Injury", photobiomodulation therapy (PBMT) in his multi-disciplinary approach particularly in regard to its remediative potential with bTBI for our combat injured Veterans.

Taking a look at emerging therapies, I can confidently predict that the 21st century will be remembered as the time when brain science truly came into its own. Broadly speaking, the first half of the 20th century was the age of psychotherapy, psychoanalysis and other talking therapies.

Following that, the second half of the 20th century was the age of pharmaceuticals and psychiatric drugs. It was from this era that the popular belief arose that by "popping pills," many disorders of the mind could be fixed. Even today anti-depressants, anti-psychotics, anxiolytics and sleeping pills are some of the most oft-prescribed medications in the Western world.

My own area of interest in this new 21st century is (photobiomodulation) PBMT, which is usually carried out by shining low-intensity near-infrared (NIR) light through the skull or through the nasal passage. These procedures are considered to be completely harmless and without any known side-effects.

One of the most important concepts that has arisen in this emerging field of neuroscience is called "synaptic plasticity", or the formation of new or strengthened connections between already existing neurons. This neuroplasticity is hypothesized to be the basis for learning and memory, especially when it occurs in the hippocampus (part of the limbic system in the brain particularly involved in memory).

In this sense, acoustical neuromodulation and photobiomodulation share a common mechanistic foundation resting on neuroplasticity. As I read about the applications of RESET Therapy to the PTSD comorbid conditions enumerated in this book, I was struck with an awareness of the inherent potential in each and every cell in our body to heal and restore itself.

When cells receive the right trigger, they are able to protect and defend us at whatever price is required. Whether the cells are stimulated by growth inducing light (PBMT) or freed from their defensive/protective mode through a healing sound (RESET), they will revert once again to a growth mode.

It is tempting to hypothesize that all of these physical interventions have mechanistic aspects in common. One of the themes unifying many apparently unrelated physical brain therapies is the upregulation of neurotrophins that support the growth, survival, and differentiation of both developing and mature neurons. An important example is brain-derived neurotrophic factor (BDNF).

Increased brain expression of BDNF has been shown to occur after PBMT as well as through aerobic exercise. I can imagine that the same effect is triggered through the effects of binaural sound. In addition to BDNF being involved in synaptogenesis, is also involved in the process of adult neurogenesis, which is the *de novo* production of newly formed neurons arising from progenitor cells in the hippocampus and sub-ventricular zone.

Dr. Margaret Naeser working with chronic TBI patients has found that some intrinsic brain networks are beneficially affected by PBMT. These networks consist of the default mode network (active during day-dreaming), the salience network (responsible for discriminating between emotional and sensory inputs), and the executive control network (responsible for decision making) all of which are positively affected by NIR light.

I personally believe that photobiomodulation is one of the most versatile and multi-faceted examples of physical brain therapies. PBMT combines some of the features of non-invasive brain stimulation techniques (resulting in increased BDNF, more synaptogenesis and neurogenesis), but also has many other relevant features which are almost unique.

However, as I read his material, it is clear that Dr. Lindenfeld has found that acoustical neuro-modulation interrupts the memory reconsolidation process within the retention network of the brain thereby permitting it to reset to pre-trauma levels. He proposes that when we combine the treatment he calls RESET Therapy with Photobiomodulation we emerge with a perfectly balanced, 'peanut-butter and jelly sandwich.'

The concept here is that intervention with RESET blocks the insidious effects of unresolved trauma from perpetuating damage to the body as a whole. On the other hand, PBMT triggers: an increase in regional cerebral blood flow; improves brain oxygenation; increases ATP levels that are crucial for effective brain function. It should be remembered that although the brain is only 5% of the total body weight, it consumes 20% of the body's supplies of glucose and oxygen.

Apparently, one shared function of both the light that induces photobiomodulation, and the sound that returns the cell to its inherent growth potential, is their apparent ability to diminish the neuro-inflammation effect. This phenomenon is especially damaging to the brain if excessively prolonged. The microglia (macrophage-like cells) within the brain respond by changing their phenotype from a pro-inflammatory activated state to an anti-inflammatory (M2) phenotype.

Incidentally it is possible that these M2 microglia are much better at phagocytosis and disposal of aggregated proteins such as the β-amyloid plaques seen in Alzheimer's disease, and the α-synuclein aggregates seen in Parkinson's disease, which might explain the particular effectiveness of PBMT in these diseases.

I look forward to what a 'peanut-butter and jelly sandwich' might offer to those who suffer from the emotional effects of trauma as well as the insidious effects of brain diseases. Perhaps this gustatory treat can be nurturing to the soul as well as to the body.

In the memorable phrase that formed the title of Dr. Lindenfeld's previous book, "Brain on Fire", it is clear that PTSD goes beyond simple "fear extinction" that has long been studied in animal models. There is a consensus that the amygdala is involved, but the hippocampus, and the ventromedial prefrontal cortex have also been implicated.

Since PBMT and acoustical neuro-modulation can both activate and deactivate networks in the brain, it would be tempting to hypothesize that fMRI could allow visualization of deactivation occurring in the amygdala after PBMT and/or RESET. It should be noted that PBMT has also been reported to decrease perception of pain, and to improve both the length and quality of sleep.

Both of these benefits might be expected to be particularly important in PTSD patients. I hope that Dr. Lindenfeld can continue to push the frontiers forward in PTSD therapy, and I personally wish him the best of luck.

Thank you, Dr. Lindenfeld,

Michael R Hamblin, Ph.D.
Wellman Center for Photomedicine
Massachusetts General Hospital
Harvard Medical School

Acknowledgement:

I appreciate and thank my colleagues who contributed clinical material that so enriched this book. As you are well aware, the topic of comorbid conditions is quite extensive with professionals specializing in perhaps only one area such as addiction throughout their entire professional career. Without their contributions, the writing of this book would not have been possible.

I thank each volunteer who agreed to contribute their experiential story in order to help others. Your contribution allowed me to explore uncertain territory in my quest to bring wholeness to those who crossed my professional threshold. I thank my family, fellow Veterans and all those who exposed their emotional wounds to me through our sharing of experiences.

Some special people are to be singled out for their efforts including my colleague, L Richard Bruursema, for his advice, expertise and overall support; Dr. Frank Lawlis for developing the primary treatment protocol and to his ongoing commitment to ending PTSD suffering in our Veterans; Dr. James C.

Miller, a psycho-physiologist and Vietnam Veteran for his vast editing expertise, physiological knowledge and all around assistance; Dr. Michael Hamblin, for bringing me into the world of light. Also, my expression of gratitude to my wife Ann, who put up with me and my fixation on this project each and every day.

Introduction:

I begin this introduction with a description of Systems Theory taken from my search efforts. I do this because I fully believe that the time has come for us to look at the effects of PTSD/trauma through a gestalt rather than a microscopic lens. The following resource was utilized for this purpose: http://www.mentalhealth andillness.com/systemstheory.html.

"All things can be viewed as a system and/or as part of a system . . . All are interconnected and affect other systems to varying degrees. All systems are constantly changing and are in dynamic balance with each other.

Systems theory summarizes concepts that apply to all systems. The proof is self-evident from observation and testing the applicability of systems theory to all systems. Systems theory is useful when approaching complex problems. . . Systems theory is quite logical and is compatible with our experience; however, it can be neither proven nor disproved by the traditional scientific method.

Systems have evolved over a dimension of time. . . The combination of a systems and evolutionary approach allows us to organize current information in a much more efficient manner. Such an approach is equally effective for astrophysics, biology, psychology, sociology etc.

To acquire a valid theory of human functioning we need to understand observations of human functioning in relation to internal and external systems. An understanding of systems theory, history and the specifics of any given system allow us to understand and therefore better predict the outcome of an event. Even with such an approach, there are limits to our ability to understand and predict.

. . . Since systems are very complex and impacted by an infinite number of other systems, we can never attain total predictability of effects. Such a view is an open systems model. In contrast, a closed system model assumes that everything does not affect everything, there are a finite number of variables that impact an outcome, and therefore, outcome is totally predictable.

An open system model still affords us some capacity to predict. We can create a hierarchy of the system variables that appear to have greatest impact upon an event. When we organize these variables, it improves our statistical capacity to predict although we are never able to attain total predictability.

. . . If those involved in problem solving remain open-minded and use an open, multi-system approach, we can benefit from others' perspectives and expertise. Occasionally, however, some use a closed system, a rigid, dogmatic approach to complex issues with the view that absolute truths and predictability exist.

Although simple solutions to complex problems are initially comforting, they prevent us from being open to the full complexity of any given problem and may cause problems that are even more complex."

I have noted in the introduction section of my earlier book (*Brain On Fire: A Therapist's Guide to Extinguishing the Flames of PTSD*) that the treatment provided to our returning Veterans for the trauma they experienced is shockingly inadequate. Looking at varied comorbid conditions that affect our aging Veterans, I can now also come to a similar conclusion.

The preponderance of our theories developed in the late 1800's and based on psychoneurotic causation now seems to be the wrong key to unlock the puzzle of PTSD. Obviously, I believe that a systems approach utilizing emerging neuroscientific information will provide the correct key.

To be more specific, I believe that we have a number of keys that are effective but we continue to cling to methods that are allegedly 'peer reviewed' and 'scientifically validated.' I question this belief with a simple challenge: Show me the cessation of the comorbid sleep disorder condition such as insomnia or nightmares associated with PTSD to back up the claim of effectiveness of the treatment approach.

One of my colleagues recently introduced me to a book entitled *Memory Reconsolidation in Psychotherapy: The Neuropsychotherapist Special Issue (1)*. Dr. Bruce Ecker's introductory description of the natural consolidation process of emotional memories eloquently conveys what I have struggled to express in my previous books. He tells us that:

"Unfading across the decades, emotional learnings display an inherent tenacity that is the bane of psychotherapists and their clients, yet this extraordinary durability appears to be a survival-positive result of natural selection, which crafted the brain such that any learning that occurs in the presence of strong emotion . . . become locked into subcortical implicit memory circuits by special synapses.

And it appears that natural selection had not created a key for that synaptic lock. . . neuroscientists have concluded by 1989 that the consolidation of learning in emotional memory was a one-way street, making consolidated learning indelible, unerasable, for the life time of the individual.

Acquired emotional responses could certainly be suppressed temporarily in various ways, . . . However, the research has shown that such counteractive measures do not actively dissolve or erase the original, problematic emotional learning. Rather, they only create a second, preferred learning that competes against and can regulate or override an unwanted response under ideal conditions, but usually not for long under real-life conditions. Relapses are almost inevitable, particularly in new or stressful situations. No wonder why therapists and clients often feel they are struggling against some unrelenting but invisible force.

. . . It is now clear that the consolidation of emotional memory is not, as had been believed for a century, a one time, final process, and that emotional memories are not indelible. Rather, neural circuits, encoding and emotional memory can be returned to a de-consolidated state, allowing erasure by new learning before a relocking-or reconsolidation-takes place."

I am basically in agreement with Dr. Ecker with one exception. It has been my experience that when the trauma involved circuitry is reset, the system 'reboots' to its pre-trauma state. This is not a new learning process but rather, an instinctive alteration from a defensive protective mode to that of a growth focus. In order to accomplish this seeming miracle, a therapist must learn the skillset necessary to develop and facilitate the change process.

As I've stated in my earlier book, let me point out that you will require both the theoretical understanding provided in this and my prior book as well as practical hands-on experience to truly become a skilled and certified provider of RESET Therapy. I am currently in the process of designing workshop formats with CEU's that will lead to your ultimate certification in this treatment procedure.

When you have developed the skills that result in a complete healing of mind, body and spirit of your patient/client, there will be no remaining doubt in your mind that finally, there is a transformative treatment that really works for PTSD and so many other conditions.

Chapter One:

Dementia

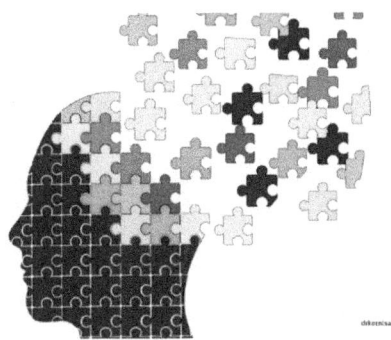

"You spend your life hoarding memories
against the day you'll lack the energy to go out and
make new ones, because that's the comfort of the old
age. The ability to look back at your life and know
that you left your mark on the world.
But I'm losing my memories, it's like someone's
broken into my piggy bank
and is robbing me one penny at a time.
It's happening so slowly,
I can hardly tell what's missing."

Shaun David Hutchinson

I hold the perspective that PTSD is one facet of a systemic disorder that affects the body and mind in a chronic and progressively destructive manner. A systemic condition affects the body in a holistic manner as opposed to a specific symptom complex perceived to be solely psychological in nature.

Partially, my viewpoint emanates from prior training in Systems Family Therapy where I was taught to look at the interactive patterns between members of a family rather than focusing only on the words they said to each other. Terms such as triangulation, hierarchical organization, boundary keeping, etc., merged with my way of thinking.

In the last few years, there has been a gradual trickle of research that is supportive of my belief that PTSD is a systemic difficulty that among other things, produces an inflammatory reaction in the brain.

To explore this hypothesis further, I co-authored a paper with Dr. George Rozelle and Dr. Katherine Billiot. We explored the hypothesis that Chronic Fatigue/Fibromyalgia is related to a brain inflammation condition as has been suggested in our earlier research with PTSD. We sought to explore if the elucidated principles would apply to CFS/FM.

Psychometric measures of the patient were taken pre- and post-treatment showing impressive statistical change. As discussed in the findings of this case study, by her fourth month of home based treatment, the patient was relatively free of CFS symptomology resulting in a significant change in her activities of daily living ("CHRONIC FATIGUE SYNDROME/ POST TRAUMATIC STRESS DISORDER,")."

I've included the topic of dementia in order to bring to your awareness recent and rather disquieting research information that I have found in 2015 – 2016 literature. The first topic is particularly startling to me in that it suggests that combat-incurred PTSD may lead to early senescence (aging) in our senior Veterans (Lohr et al,)

The second alarming finding suggests that combat veterans with PTSD are twice as likely as their non-combat colleagues to incur a dementing disorder as they age (Pinciotti et al) Yet another study of those Veterans with sleep difficulties suggested that they are 27% more likely to develop dementia as compared to their colleagues without sleep disturbance (Yaffe, et al)

Aside from the emotional change that trauma produces, investigators are now inquiring into the effect that PTSD has upon normal bodily functioning. The researchers are questioning how this change may produce physical and behavioral susceptibility in the patient.

I will address each of these issues in more detail as we proceed with this discourse. I will also include a compelling case study related to the use of RESET Therapy in a patient with documented memory difficulties found to be produced by pseudodementia.

A 2015 assessment by Lohr parallels my own conclusion that PTSD is more likely to represent a systemic condition. Lohr noted that:

"In short, evidence from multiple lines of investigation suggests that PTSD may be associated with a phenotype of accelerated senescence (aging). Further research is critical to understand the nature of this association. . . There may be a need to re-conceptualize PTSD beyond the boundaries of mental illness, and instead as a full systemic disorder." (Lohr et al., 2015)

Indeed, while studies of this type are relatively sparse in the literature, I found a 2016 analysis focused on how the later emergence of PTSD affects the aging combat Veteran and his/her caregiver. The authors noted that: "veterans with posttraumatic stress disorder (PTSD) are twice as likely as other veterans to develop dementia." (Pinciotti et al., 2016)

If this weren't enough, yet another revelation can be found in a recent 2016 study that looked at pathological markers, as assessed by amyloid and tau imaging with PET. The authors investigated whether; "Vietnam war veterans without mild cognitive impairment or dementia, but with chronic combat related PTSD show evidence of Alzheimer's disease." (AD) They found that:

Despite the PTSD cohort being significantly younger than the controls, there was a significant difference in the age-corrected ⋯ retention between the PTSD and control groups. . . Our preliminary findings suggest that chronic PTSD might be associated with higher neocortical tau deposition later in life. Further work is required to determine if chronic PTSD itself, or associated lifestyle factors account for this observation (Cummins et al., 2016)

Sleep disturbance is also a comorbid feature associated with PTSD. The authors of this study (Yaffe et al., 2015) sought to determine whether a diagnosis of sleep disturbance is associated with dementia in older veterans. They obtained medical record data from the Department of Veterans Affairs National Patient Care Database for 200,000 randomly selected veterans aged 55 years and older. The authors found that:

After adjusting for potential confounders, those with sleep disturbance had a 27% increased risk of dementia. . . Sleep disturbance was associated with increased risk of dementia among a large cohort of older, primarily male veterans. (Yaffe, Nettiksimmons, Yesavage, & Byers, 2015)

Now I personally find the above material to be staggering in its potential impact. To restate it differently, if the service member experienced combat involvement, he or she is likely to: physically age earlier; have a sleep disorder; be twice as likely to develop a dementing condition as compared to his/her service colleagues who did not engage in combat. To further complicate matters, delayed-onset post-traumatic stress disorder (DOPTSD) is evidencing itself in increasing numbers among those Veterans who have served decades ago.

The authors of the following article further note that the scars of combat experience involving trauma of various kinds apparently leave invisible wounds that do not heal. They focused on those Veterans with dementia who were placed in nursing facilities commenting that apparently, "*Bathing Without a Battle (BWOB)*, in nursing home care facilities is a relatively frequent occurrence."

This is certainly something that I haven't been aware of previously, being primarily focused on outpatient treatment settings. Nor have I been aware of the incidence of PTSD emerging in later life among those Veterans who may have evidenced the symptoms at an earlier time, but were relatively intact after the symptoms subsided. The authors note that:

". . . Many years after a war, other aging veterans find themselves fighting a new battle as they strive to cope with delayed-onset posttraumatic stress disorder." (DOPTSD)

"For many aging military veterans with Post Traumatic Stress Disorder (PTSD) activities of daily living, particularly bathing, can be an improbable, exasperating, and stressful task.

". . . The bathing process for elderly male military veterans suffering from DOPTSD is often a challenging experience for both veterans and their caregivers. Similar to dementia, persons with DOPTSD can become confused and may misinterpret actions and verbiage by caretakers." (Rose, 2015)

The preceding article was provided to illustrate some of the issues becoming evident in the aging combat Veteran population. I'm not sure if the above author is proposing that the population he is referring to is different than those diagnosed with Alzheimer's or some other form of dementia. My read is that the populations are the same.

In yet another study extracted from the National Health and Resilience in Veterans Study, the authors noted that over 60% of our Veterans are over 55 years of age and that the results of the inquiry further revealed that:

". . . 9.9% of older US veterans experienced exacerbated PTSD symptoms an average of nearly 3 decades after their worst trauma. . . Approximately 1 in 10 older US veterans experiences a clinically significant exacerbation of PTSD symptoms in late life. Executive dysfunction may contribute to risk for exacerbated PTSD symptoms. . . These results suggest that exacerbated PTSD symptoms are prevalent in US veterans and highlight potential targets for identifying veterans at risk for this phenomenon." (Mota et al., 2016)

If these figures are accurate, we need to begin planning immediately for the onslaught of those aging Veterans who will be filling our already pressed nursing homes for additional space. Alternatively, we might come to the conclusion that PTSD is indeed a systemic issue and invest in methodology to reset trauma circuitry in the brain back to its pre-trauma state.

Furthermore, we need to immediately explore methodology that can potentially reverse the onset of senescence. In a 2014 article, the authors explored a linkage between depression, trauma and dementia in the later stages of life. They suggest that:

". . . The most likely biologic mechanisms that may link depression and dementia among military veterans include vascular disease, changes in glucocorticoid steroids and hippocampal atrophy, deposition of β-amyloid plaques, inflammatory changes, and alterations of nerve growth factors. In addition, military veterans often have depression comorbid with posttraumatic stress disorder or traumatic brain injury. "Therefore, in military veterans, these hypothesized biologic pathways going from depression to dementia are more than likely influenced by trauma-related processes.

". . . Given the projected increase of dementia, as well as the projected increase in the older segment of the veteran population, in the future, it is critically important that we understand whether treatment for depression alone or combined with other regimens improves cognition." (Byers & Yaffe, 2014)

The metabolic syndrome (MetS) is a biochemical process that has been linked to the long-term effects of PTSD. Examples of this would be such conditions as diabetes and stroke. The authors of this 2016 article suggest that:

"Post-traumatic stress disorder (PTSD) is associated with elevated risk for metabolic syndrome (MetS). However, the direction of this association is not yet established, as most prior studies employed cross-sectional designs. The primary goal of this study was to evaluate bidirectional associations between PTSD and MetS using a longitudinal design.

". . . The prevalence of MetS among veterans with PTSD was just under 40% at both time points and was significantly greater than that for veterans without PTSD; the prevalence of MetS among those with PTSD was also elevated relative to age-matched population estimates. . . Results highlight the substantial cardio-metabolic concerns of young veterans with PTSD and raise the possibility that PTSD may predispose individuals to accelerated aging, in part, manifested clinically as MetS." (Wolf et al., 2016)

An earlier study (2014) examined the relationship between PTSD symptoms over the course of treatment and associated changes in general physical health symptoms. Positive health habits such as exercising and negative such as excessive eating was examined to determine if they accounted for the association between changes in PTSD severity as well as changes in physical health over time. The authors found that:

"150 women seeking treatment for PTSD revealed a substantial relationship (34%) between changes in PTSD and changes in physical health that occurred during and shortly following treatment for PTSD. However, there was no evidence to suggest that changes in health behaviors accounted for this relationship. Thus, PTSD treatment can have beneficial effects on self-reported physical health symptoms, even without direct treatment focus on health per se, and is not accounted for by shifts in health behavior." (Shipherd, Clum, Suvak, & Resick, 2014)

The authors of the following 2015 article note that PTSD is associated with high rates of obesity and cardiometabolic diseases although there are few studies that have explored this relationship. Consequently, they conducted a review of the literature (1980-2014) related to physical activity and eating behaviors in adults with PTSD or PTSD symptoms. The authors found that:

> . . . there may be a negative association among PTSD, physical activity, and eating behaviors. Preliminary evidence from 3 pilot intervention studies suggests that changes in physical activity or diet may have beneficial effects on PTSD symptoms. . . More evidence in representative samples, using multivariable analytical techniques, is needed to identify a definitive relationship between PTSD and these health behaviors. (Hall, Hoerster, & Yancy, 2015)

The term pseudo-dementia was first used in 1961 to describe cognitive deficits in depression, especially when it is found in old age (Kiloh, 1961). The authors of a 2014 study addressed the issue of diagnostic confusion between dementia and pseudo-dementia. Consequently, they reviewed scientific literature pertaining to cognitive deficits that present in this condition. They note that:

"Present review suggests that over past few decades, enough study results point to the fact that depressive states adversely affect cognitive functions, especially in old-age or geriatric depression. In spite of the methodological and sampling problems encountered when working with these complex populations, the differentiation between depression and early stages of dementia seems to be plausible.

". . . most of the recent data support this practice and should be able to differentiate between true cases of dementia, depression and the ill-defined intermediate stage of pseudo-dementia. Subsequent endeavors in this area with more well-defined populations and properly designed studies are needed to generalize these conclusions." (Kang et al., 2014)

Cohen et. al., presented a case history involving pseudodementia as a delayed traumatic stress response. The authors reported that the patient regained full functioning over the next year:

Although an organic cause could not be ruled out, it was likely that recovery of traumatic memories was contributory to the patient's condition, as ongoing psychotherapy had begun 1 year into the course. If additional cases with similar presentations are reported, such cases would corroborate the notion that persistent, severe, and reversible cognitive impairment constitutes a previously unrecognized and atypical posttraumatic response. (Cohen & Brody, 2015)

Interestingly, I encountered a similar case based on a neurological referral to neuropsychologically evaluate an 86-year-old patient. The request specified that I ascertain if dementia was the cause of her reported memory slippage. While this is a rather lengthy report, I include it to illustrate the patient's recovery from repressed traumatic experiences.

Although I'm sure that the case I will present here is not the second to be reported in the literature, I am sure that it is the first one to discuss remediation from pseudodementia through the RESET Therapy process. Because of the length of this fascinating case study, the material will not be indented.

This 86-year-old woman was born in Germany and lived through the Nazi regime before finally immigrating to the United States at age 17 with her family in 1953. Her story is one of multiple traumas, enormous courage, and an incessant desire to find personal resolution to the horrors she previously encountered.

Because of the enormity of her suffering, her mind repressed major aspects of her earlier years leading her to believe that she had amnesia for large blocks of time primarily around World War II events. This affected her memory over time leading her to seek professional assistance in an effort to remediate this condition. It was an honor to assist her in at least partially accomplishing this objective. Her story follows:

"I met Dr. Lindenfeld when the doctors were trying to figure out if I had a stroke because, I had problems with word finding with my memory. Trying to be responsible, I agreed to have neuropsychological testing provided and was quite shaken up over the fact of how great the deficits were. Tasks which I could have done previously with ease were impossible for me to now complete.

"After this testing was finished, Doctor Lindenfeld introduced me to a new experimental treatment in order to regain some of those abilities. Previous to the treatment, I had been aware that I was suffering with PTSD. I had read about soldiers with PTSD with their nightmares and other symptoms. Loud noises made me shake and the sound of airplanes caused me to become very afraid. I've had problems with my long-term memory from childhood times.

"I was born by Caesarean Section, the first performed in that particular hospital however, I was born Placenta Previa and was 4 weeks early. Both, my mother and I had lung problems and I was not expected to live. The physician recommended that as much fresh air as possible be provided for me. Even at that young age, I learned to love the healing energy of the outdoors and I became 'contemplative'. This fact helped me to survive what was yet to come in my life.

"When we got to this country, I was immature and after a failed marriage, got remarried to a psychologist at age 29. I was married to him for 10 years and was in the hospital for a tumor in my spine. He died traumatically two days after my surgery leaving me at 39 a widow with an 8-year-old child. I lived with my parents for a while and then went to nursing school. I got my RN and later my Master's degree. I worked for 31 years as a nurse.

"The doctor (Lindenfeld) introduced me to a treatment which sounded too good to be true so I went to the first session a little skeptical, but desperate to find help. To my amazement, I went immediately into an early experience I witnessed as a child of a gruesome treatment received by a Russian captive by German SS soldiers stomping him with their Nazi boots.

"I heard harsh swear words in German (schweinhunt) recalling this in my native language. It brought memories back to me of a time that I had long forgotten and apparently repressed from the ages of 5 to 13. It brought back the memories of something that had been in the back of my mind and had brought nightmares to me for years.

"I found myself as a child hanging onto a staircase secretly watching while this abuse occurred and then the fear faded away into the pulsing sound coming from the treatment device. I recalled that the Nazi found a Russian prisoner hiding in the basement of our house. I remembered the sound of the screaming as they repeatedly kicked him.

"After each treatment, I felt relieved and lighter in spirit and it encouraged me to seek additional sound treatment for other war experiences in my life. With the first treatment, I remembered everything from that event with no emotional content lingering after I left the office.

"I experienced some nausea which is typical for me when I tend to worry. I talked with my son about what occurred which is unusual for me. In my second treatment, I found it to be a lot worse than I thought it would be. I could hear the machine gun fire and land mines going off and the screams so clearly all around me. I was totally in the sounds of death. It was truly a miracle that my family was able to make it out.

"After, the second treatment, I was amazed that I was able to regain the memory and not the emotional content. Also, stuff keeps coming up for me. I learned very early to disassociate. I would go into the light when I felt threatened. There, I would feel safe. My brother would say that I had one foot on a banana and the other in heaven.

"I see light around people – the essence of the being. With negative – the light is interrupted and goes closer to the body. I would go into the light when I felt threatened. I'm feeling lighter now. I had time after the last session when there was joy. I feel it now. It's been years since I felt it.

"The last forty to fifty years there's been only anxiety and depression. After the treatments, I felt hopeful again. The final treatment that I asked the doctor to provide me with was the continuing nightmare about the wall falling in on me. I have received that final treatment and now I'm free of it at last.

"I remember so many things that I thought were gone from me. The doctor said that two types of RESET were used to free these memories from my mind including the PTSD and Depression ones. Here is my story that I now can share with you fully and completely.

"My family were large scale farmers and land owners in Sterbenien, East Germany located near the Polish border. On my mother's side, there were pastors who were friends with Martin Luther and they published some papers.

"Another part of the family included an opera singer who lived with us and she was very close to me. I remember that she played the piano and I'd hide under it and listen to the music. Frequently, she would interrupt playing and just look at me and smile. There was a gong for certain meals and sometimes we would go to the meal and sometimes we would not.

"The house we lived in was four stories tall. I had four siblings and we were close because of the class system in the village. The villagers were reticent to let their children play with us because my father was the owner of the village and the farms around them. They looked up to him and my mother but there was still a class system separation between the workers and the owners.

"I was born in 1935 at a time when things started to heat up in Germany. When Hitler came to power everything changed including the commerce. My father used to export seed potatoes and grains to Italy which became no longer possible. When the war had started, airplanes would fly over our estate and there were battles in the sky above us. The only place we could hide was in a ditch dug by the workers.

"There were several planes that were shot down and whoever was in the plane died. At that time, the pogroms started in Poland and in particular, the Jewish synagogues were destroyed. My mother organized the village women and there were men and women who worked with the resistance who told us about destruction of the temples and killing of the Jewish communities.

"My mother let it be known that she would shelter and feed people and they started coming in around 1940. At first, they were scattered but then regular refugee lines formed around us. They were stunned, had very little facial expression and their clothes were torn and tattered. Especially in the winter, when it was cold, they had frozen feet and hands.

"Because there was always fear of someone informing about this, they could only stay a night or at most, two nights with us. I recall this going on for two years until the German SS soldiers took occupation of the village. The commandant lived in our house with us. It was difficult for the refugees to come to our farm and many of them were killed on the highway.

"My aunt refused to do the "Heil Hitler" saying that, "the next regime will come in and ask me to raise my leg." We were very young at the time and we had certain places in the house where we could hide. It was pretty much a grim existence because of the occupation.

"When the warfront moved into where we lived due to the Russian advance, some of the American and "British airplanes would bomb the cities. We had two bombs that exploded in the field nearby. For a while, the soldiers left the village again in 1943 and we had more refugees coming in.

"My father was told that they were going to arrest him and my mother as well as the children and he already has started to prepare wagons for our flight. He constructed the wagons pretty much like the pioneers did here.

"Our Persian rugs were put over the wagons to keep the wind out. When we heard machine-gun fire and bombs landing near us, we had to leave. My father heard from an informant that they were coming to arrest him.

"It was winter and about thirty degrees below zero when we got into the wagons. Some of the villagers came with us. The schoolteacher was picked up in a coach and there was no time for him and his wife to transfer to a wagon.

"The fields were frozen and my father drove the horses across the fields because the Germans and the Russians were on the highway or on the roads. We had to keep the horses moving so that their hoofs wouldn't freeze to the ground. We were separated from the teacher and we don't know if he survived or not.

"We saw one man who walked dazed on the road and my mother recognized him as one of the Jewish refugees. He was part of the group of about sixty refugees and was the only survivor. During the trip, we were advancing with the German Army when we could, but again my father had to lead the horses. At one time the wind blew the cover off the wagon and I looked out and saw the head of a small child with a drop of blood on the cheek like a tear.

"I've had that nightmare many times. The sounds around me were horrendous. The machine guns, other guns and the sound of men and women dying were all consuming. Some of the fleeing Germans thought they should wear their uniform. The Russians would arrest them and hang them. As we rode in the wagons down the road I could see the corpses of German refugees that had put on a uniform.

"Instead of going west, we went east towards Gdansk because my father's uncle was part of the German occupation and he could get us on a boat to cross by sea and not go by land. These boats were to be provided for the German soldiers who were retreating.

"On the road, my father traded some food for a map of the surrounding minefields. When there was an explosion and light flared up, he would walk the horses across the field. Before we got into the town of Gdansk we had to leave the wagons and my parents and five of us kids and a driver were stuffed into a Volkswagen. My father had to take his warm coat off in order to fit in.

"The driver took us to the boat and we boarded. When we left the harbor, we had U-boats that were escorting us and we lost them in a heavy fog. The captain made everyone put on a life vest and my parents bound us together with a rope so that if the boat went under, we would be together. By this point, the children and my parents looked the same as the Jewish refugees - stunned and without expression. The fight was going on the ground and in the air but the boat was able to get beyond the battle zone.

"The children and my mother ended up on an island called Ru'gen where we stayed with my mother's sister. My father was drafted to the city of Hamburg in West Germany forcing us to be apart for a year. Before the Russians left, they would come silently to the island and capture the women and rape them. For us children, we had the task of warning the women when the Russians were coming.

"The Russians came to the house where we stayed and they took all the furniture. When my mother complained, they said you are lucky that you have your head. At that point, the Cossack's part of the Russian army came in and took charge of the island.

"They were beautiful to see on white horses and they did not rape or plunder. My mother said that I was raped and stabbed by the Russians. She said that I was stabbed in the belly. I've kinda pushed this awareness away all my life.

"Essentially, someone told my mother that the Russians were putting the refugees from the East into a train to the camps in Russia/Siberia. My mother packed all we could carry and we walked seven miles on a bridge from the island to the mainland. East German police helped my mother to jump a freight train which was filled with refugees from Berlin.

"They were very angry and threatened to throw us off the train because we didn't have a pink slip. In this whole time, I withdrew into myself and saw light that surrounded me that I believed would keep me safe. I had the experience before when I was a young child, that I saw light around people, animals and trees, anything living.

"There were about 60 people in this freight car and no restroom facilities. My mother had a chamber pot for my younger sister and it became a ticket to freedom. It was handed around to people who needed it and a German soldier who was at the door had to keep emptying it making jokes about it.

"When we came near the border, where the Iron Curtain was, the train stopped and we heard doors of the freight cars being opened and screaming people loaded into trucks. My mother told the people who were still trying to get rid of us that if we could not all be silent, we would be part of the people taken to Russia.

"It did get very quiet and for the first time, I heard people praying. My light grew to encompass most of the freight car. I was a little upset about that because it was my light and it shouldn't shelter them. When the Russians came down the line of the freight train, they got into an argument in front of our car and forgot to open the door. The freight train then continued into the Western zone that included the British and American zone.

"We were taken off the train and put into a refugee camp which had tents with straw on the floor and each family got a little corner of that. We all had to go through shower rooms naked and got sprayed with delousing material and got some clothing to put on and we stayed in the camp for two nights.

"American soldiers were very kind to us. They gave children candy and one man gave my mother a carton of Camel cigarettes. She later bartered those to get tickets on the train to the town of Hamburg where my father was supposed to be. We eventually arrived at the train station in Hamburg. We later found out that my father had made several attempts to cross the Iron Curtain to get to us but had been unsuccessful.

"The streets of Hamburg were nothing like my mother remembered. It was mostly bombed out and we had to walk over many obstacles. We arrived at the apartment where we thought my father lived, who at that time was living with my mother's brother and his wife and daughter. We were there for several months.

"My father was working for a lumber company and he would bring home a backpack of wood every night and trade it on the black market for food. We were stationed in a refugee camp near the town of Wilhelmshafen. My father worked in the administration office and my mother ran the laundry.

"Among the refugees was a schoolteacher who organized the children in these difficult times. With little food, we always felt a little lightheaded and the teacher had been a heavy smoker and had to live without any cigarettes. My parents were in the same boat. Most of the adults smoked. Some tried to make cigarettes out of rose petals and newspapers.

"Because of this general condition, the adults were short tempered. We were housed in barracks with primitive facilities. There was no electricity or light in the evening. We lit a candle in order to do our homework. Our lunch usually consisted of a slice of rutabaga and we would fantasize about all different kinds of delicious sandwiches.

"There was a pastor among the refugees who prepared those of us who are old enough for the service of confirmation. He had services in a bombed-out church that was supported by planks. When we were lined up for confirmation some of the supports broke and the wall came down.

"My best friend was next to me and I was holding her hand. Eventually her hand got cold and I knew she was dead. I heard a lot of noises and people removing parts of the wall, trying to lift up the wooden supports. At first, I pleaded with God to save me and then I got angry and I thought that if this is the kind of God that you are, I don't want to know you.

"At some point, I must've fallen asleep and when I opened my eyes, I saw the light again. In my anger, I did not connect the light with the God who is merciful. I just was comforted by the light. One of the wooden supports was pressing down on my back and the pain was at times, unbearable. I called for help but in the general noise, couldn't hear anybody responding. At some point, just before the rescue, the wall shifted and made the pain much worse.

"At some point, I lost consciousness and when I came to, I was being attended to by paramedics. Since that time, in my dreams I repeated the scenes of terror and fear because I didn't know if anyone was helping. This has gone on for sixty-six years. Now the dreams are gone. My last treatment focused on this terror and now, I am finally free of it. (11/2014)

"For several years, my mother and father managed a shelter for elderly refugees from Russia, Estonia, Latvia etc. There they met a Lutheran pastor from Saginaw, Michigan, who offered to sponsor us for coming to the U.S. and finally, by 1953, we had all the necessary papers in order.

"When we reached Ellis Island my older brother had a high fever. Fortunately, my mother was able to bring his temperature down with cold packs and aspirin and we were able to pass and did not have to stay on Ellis Island. On Feb. 1953, we arrived in New York. I had difficulties adjusting to the culture of poodle skirts and bobby sox and saddle shoes in High School.

"I was 17 years old and was used to serious study in a Liberal Arts track in the Gymnasium in Germany. I had appeared in some plays and sang in a radio children's choir during that time. The King's English that I had learned previously was not very helpful to understand the other students at the High School I attended in Saginaw, Michigan. This began my life long struggle with poor self-esteem.

"After graduation, I worked as an apprentice at a Summer-stock Theater where I met my first husband who was the art director. He was 32 years old and I was 18 when we married. I had no idea that he was gay, nor did I know what homosexuality was. When I finally discovered that he was an active homosexual, I sought therapy assistance after speaking to my physician who referred me to a psychotherapist.

"Through talk therapy, I attained clarification regarding what homosexuality was and the impact that this would have on my life. People in my immediate family raised questions as to whether a homosexual would be able to properly assist me in raising the four boys that we had together.

"I really loved the man and had I been more enlightened, in retrospect, I would have stayed with him and worked it out. I continued in therapy for a while and eventually saw a psychiatrist who prescribed me with antidepressant medication.

"Two of my children had learning disabilities and I was referred to a psychologist who specialized in this area. The therapist worked with the children and over time became more and more involved until eventually, we began to date and ultimately married when I was 35.

"I've always been over reactive to stress believing that this was connected to my wartime experience in Germany. I was told by doctors that this was due to my unrealistic reaction to stress with the onus always placed on me as a patient and not the inadequacy of the treatment or the medication. Always, the prescribed medication I was provided didn't work well however, I continued to take it as prescribed.

"Eventually, my husband insisted that I see a psychologist again and I proceeded to reengage in therapy where I came to realize that my husband was experiencing many mental problems himself. After discussing this with him, he was opposed to addressing this through any form of therapeutic intervention. He was particularly concerned with people being after him and when he came home from the hospital, I would sit up with him to assist him to process his concerns.

"Being of the Jewish extraction, he was persecuted as a child in school because of this and still the fear continued throughout his life's experiences. In the meantime, I was dealing with my children and he really didn't want to get involved in their upbringing. The raising of the children and household was all put upon me.

"When I was with him, I joined the Church of Christ and he became the head of the congregation. I think that his conversion from Judaism bothered him a lot so I had to support him in his role by participating in meetings with the pastor. One day the pastor came to me to talk about church related issues however, he proceeded to rape me.

"I remember getting very nervous and having anger because I didn't know how to deal with it. Again, I went to the psychiatrist and got yet another medication because my husband had a certain standing in the church community. It always seemed that it was my fault when things didn't go right such as the medications provided to me not having a good effect.

"My husband wouldn't confront the pastor and we left the church. This proceeded to haunt me as long as I was married to him. Eventually, I stopped participating in therapy due to financial reasons. I stayed with the medication for a while but eventually stopped that too because I felt better without it.

"In 1976 we ultimately divorced because of incompatibility. For me, it was financially difficult because he would contribute to the household but not to the education of my children. I became involved in nursing and obtained a degree in 1975. I pursued a master's degree in nursing and completed that in 1980. In the meantime, I felt bad about not being there for my children but did make an effort to be there for them when they came home from school.

"In the late 80s, I saw a psychologist who focused on Reiki Body Focused Therapy. Through this intervention, I came to realize that I was suffering with the effects of PTSD. I didn't feel that I was doing a good job with this intervention and did not really see any improvement of my symptoms and, in fact, the symptomatology worsened.

"I had periods of breaking out in tears and would be unable to be physically present for my children when this occurred. I finally got another medication which made me numb thereby permitting me to do my day to day activity as a nurse in the intensive care setting.

"In 1984, I again engaged in therapy because of the ongoing nightmares and inability to sleep due to flashbacks to the war experiences. The psychologist provided me with EMDR treatment which helped me to do my day work but, it didn't stop the flashbacks and nightmares. From that point, I lived with my life through developing my spirituality to help me to cope with what ailed me.

"Finally, with RESET therapy, after all this time, the nightmares are gone but I still have memories which come up. I am able to deal with them because I no longer panic. Now, it's like reading a book. When I had them before, my hands would start shaking and I'd be close to tears but that doesn't happen anymore. Finally, I'm free of the effects of that horrible time in my life."

Summary

The concept of PTSD as a systemic difficulty was introduced with a small number of supportive controlled studies purporting this point of view. In fact, I added the first chapter due to disquieting and disturbing findings emerging from my recent review of scientific literature related to the aging process in our senior Veterans.

The data suggests that our Veterans continue to cumulate the effects of earlier service-incurred traumas even though obvious symptoms of PTSD are not evident. As they age, the symptoms manifest as prefrontal lobe control weakens over the course of time. If these findings prove to be valid, we are potentially facing a tsunami of demand from our aging Veterans: one that our current support system is simply incapable of providing.

Alternatively, as you will uncover within this book, a straight-forward non-invasive intervention can stop the procession of the PTSD aspect. Furthermore, as you will read in the next chapter, a treatment referred to as Photobiomodulation is offering the potential for reversing the effects of dementia as well as traumatic brain injury in those afflicted with this dual disturbance.

The topic of pseudo-dementia was introduced due to my experience as a former evaluating psychologist. I've been involved with numerous cases that were thought to be Alzheimer's or some other form of dementia. Ultimately, a number of these cases proved to be directly related to earlier traumas and were shown to be reversible with the proper treatment intervention.

This might lead one to ask how many of our Veterans are misdiagnosed and provided with medications that don't address the underlying difficulties? How many of them could experience a reversal of what is expected to be an ever-increasing decline of mental capacity as they age?

The lengthy and compelling case study I earlier provided exemplifies the above circumstances. I'm sure each generation holds the view that we live in exciting times. I can certainly say this within the context of my own life's experiences as related to the application of RESET Therapy.

Reference List:

Byers, A. L., & Yaffe, K. (2014). Depression and dementias among military veterans. *Alzheimer's & Dementia: The Journal of the Alzheimer's Associa tion, 10*(3 Suppl), S166-173. https://doi.org/ 10.1016/ j.jalz.2014.04.007

CHRONIC FATIGUE SYNDROME/POST TRAUMATIC STRESS DISORDER: ARE THEY ALIKE? https://www.academia .edu/27251041/ CH-RONIC_FATIGUE_SYNDROME_POST_T RAUMATIC_STRESS_DISORDER_ARE_T HEY_ALIKE

CHRONIC_FATIGUE.docx. (n.d.). Retrieved from http://s3.amazonaws.com/academia.edu.docu ments/47510366/CHRONIC_FATIGUE.docx ?AWSAccessKeyId=AKIAJ56TQJRTWSMT NPEA&Expires=1471423100&Signature=6Z AjPOd26zGqjY4s5LXvzF5f8gE%3D&respo

nse-content-disposition=attachment%
3B%20filename%3DCHRONIC_FATIGUE_
SYNDROME_POST_TRAUMATIC.docx

Cohen, L. J., & Brody, D. (2015). Frontotemporal
Dementia-Like Syndrome Following Recall
of Childhood Sexual Abuse. *Journal of
Traumatic Stress, 28*(3), 240–246.
https://doi.org/10.1002 /jts.22016

Cummins, T., Elias, A., Hopwood, M., Rosenfeld, J.,
DorÃ©, V., Lamb, F., ... Rowe, C. (2016).
Assessing Aβ & tau pathology in Vietnam
war veterans with chronic Post-Traumatic
Stress Disorder. *Journal of Nuclear Medicine,
57*(supplement 2), 1230–1230.

Johnstone, D. M., Moro, C., Stone, J., Benabid, A.-
L., & Mitrofanis, J. (2016). Turning On
Lights to Stop Neurodegeneration: The
Potential of Near Infrared Light Therapy in
Alzheimer's and Parkinson's Disease.
Frontiers in Neuroscience, 9. https://doi.org
/10.3389/fnins.2015.00500

Kang, H., Zhao, F., You, L., Giorgetta, C., D, V.,
Sarkhel, S., & Prakash, R. (2014). Pseudo-
dementia: A neuropsychological review.
*Annals of Indian Academy of Neurology,
17*(2), 147–154. https://doi
.org/10.4103/0972-2327.132613

Kiloh, L. G. (1961). Pseudo-Dementia. *Acta
Psychiatrica Scandinavica, 37*(4), 336–351.

https://doi.org/10.1111/j.1600-0447.1961
.tb07367.x

Lohr, J. B., Palmer, B. W., Eidt, C. A., Aailaboyina,
S., Mausbach, B. T., Wolkowitz, O. M., …
Jeste, D. V. (2015). Is Post-Traumatic Stress
Disorder Associated with Premature
Senescence? A Review of the Literature. *The
American Journal of Geriatric Psychiatry:
Official Journal of the American Association
for Geriatric Psychiatry*, *23*(7), 709–725.
https://doi.org/10.1016/j.jagp.2015.04.001

Mota, N., Tsai, J., Kirwin, P. D., Harpaz-Rotem, I.,
Krystal, J. H., Southwick, S. M., & Pietrzak,
R. H. (2016). Late-life exacerbation of PTSD
symptoms in US veterans: results from the
National Health and Resilience in Veterans
Study. *The Journal of Clinical Psychiatry*,
77(3), 348–354. https://doi.org/10.4088
/JCP.15m10101

Pinciotti, C. M., Bass, D. M., McCarthy, C. A.,
Judge, K. S., Wilson, N. L., Morgan, R. O.,
… Kunik, M. E. (2016). Negative
Consequences of Family Caregiving for
Veterans With PTSD and Dementia: *The
Journal of Nervous and Mental Disease*, 1.
https://doi.org/10.1097/NMD
.0000000000000560

Purushothuman, S., Johnstone, D. M., Nandasena, C.,
Eersel, J. van, Ittner, L. M., Mitrofanis, J., &
Stone, J. (2015). Near infrared light mitigates

cerebellar pathology in transgenic mouse models of dementia. *Neuroscience Letters, 591*, 155–159. https://doi.org /10.1016/ j.neulet.2015.02.037

Rose, M. (2015). Fighting a New Battle: A Bathing Care Standard for Caregivers of Elderly Male Military Veterans with Delayed Onset Post Traumatic Stress Disorder. Presented at the 43rd Biennial Convention (07 November - 11 November 2015), STTI. https://stti.confex. com/stti/bc43/ webprogram/Paper74013.html

Salgado, A. S. I., Zângaro, R. A., Parreira, R. B., & Kerppers, I. I. (2015). The effects of transcranial LED therapy (TCLT) on cerebral blood flow in the elderly women. *Lasers in Medical Science, 30*(1), 339–346. https://doi. org/10.1007/s10103-014-1669-2

Yaffe, K., Nettiksimmons, J., Yesavage, J., & Byers, A. (2015). Sleep Quality and Risk of Dementia Among Older Male Veterans. *The American Journal of Geriatric Psychiatry: Official Journal of the American Association for Geriatric Psychiatry, 23*(6), 651–654. https://doi.org/10.1016-/j.jagp.2015.02.008

Chapter Two:

TRAUMATIC BRAIN INJURY

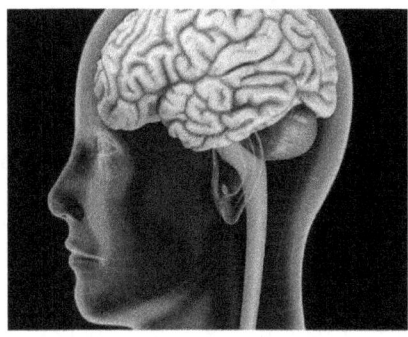

"Even in times of trauma, we try to maintain a sense of normality until we no longer can. That, my friends, is called surviving. Not healing. We never become whole again ... we are survivors. If you are here today... you are a survivor. But those of us who have made it thru hell and are still standing? We bare a different name: warriors."

Lori Goodwin

In my book, *Brain On Fire: A Therapist's Guide to Extinguishing the Flames of PTSD*, I included a chapter entitled: The Hidden Wound. My plan in this chapter is to build on what was provided in the earlier book. I intend to provide you with a foundation of understanding related to a newly emerging science that offers the potential for at least partial remediation of traumatic brain injury as well as dementing disorders such as Alzheimer's Disease.

However, before discussing incidence rates and an impressive emerging treatment, let's take a look at a case example provided in a 2005 New England Journal of Medicine article in order to be able to fully appreciate the life altering consequences of a bTBI wound:

"Sergeant David Emme, a supply officer with a U.S. Army Stryker Brigade, was stationed at a submachine gun on a truck rolling through northern Iraq last November, in a convoy transporting Iraqi volunteers to Mosul for military training. As they entered the town of Talafar, Emme noticed that the streets were unusually quiet: no children were outdoors running toward the vehicles demanding sweets.

"Emme got on the radio and warned others in the convoy: "Something might happen. They might have some plan for us." Moments later, as they slowed at a traffic circle, an improvised explosive device (IED) went off right next to Emme's truck, knocking him out.

". . . I remember waking up and wondering who the hell I was, where the hell I was, and why can't I see or hear? My soldier was screaming for me to get out of the truck and I told him no, because it hurt too much. So he literally threw me out of the truck and guided me to a Stryker, a lightweight armored vehicle."

"The blast wave and fragments from the explosion had blown out Emme's left eardrum, fractured his skull, injured his left eye, and caused a severe contusion in the left frontotemporal area of his brain. His fellow soldiers rushed him to the nearby military base, where he partially regained his vision and tried to walk before again losing consciousness.

". . . neurosurgeons performed a craniectomy, removing a large piece of skull from the left temporal region to give Emme's brain room to swell. In the five months since then, Emme, 32, has made a remarkable recovery from his severe brain injury. . .

"His vision has returned almost to normal. With time and intensive therapy, his speech and cognitive function have dramatically improved. "Basically, I had to learn what things were again," Emme explained. Then he corrected himself: "I knew what they were — I just didn't know what the names of them were." (Okie, 2005)

A 2014 study investigated military Veterans exposed to mild TBIs as compared to a Veteran group with no TBI exposure and a civilian group with no history of concussion. The researchers sought evidence of detectible indicators through a variety of interventions including: multiple neuroimaging modalities, neuro-psychologic evaluation; cerebrospinal fluid (CSF) analysis. The authors commented that:

"Traumatic brain injury (TBI) is the best-established risk factor for Alzheimer's disease (AD) in late life. Repetitive mild TBIs, "concussions," can produce chronic traumatic encephalopathy (CTE, the former "dementia puglistica") with tau-containing neuro-fibrillary tangles histologically indistinguishable from AD.

"Given that mild TBI from explosive blast is the "signature injury" of the wars in Iraq and Afghanistan, we asked if combat Veterans who had experienced repetitive mild TBIs in these conflicts demonstrated structural and/or functional brain abnormalities on four neuroimaging modalities, subtle cognitive impairment on neuropsychologic evaluation, or neurodegeneration biomarkers in cerebrospinal fluid (CSF).

"Subjects included a deployed Veteran group with a history of blast concussion mild TBI (n=54); a deployed Veteran group with no (lifetime) history of TBI (n=25); and civilian controls with no history of concussion (n=67).

"Years after returning from combat deployments in Iraq and Afghanistan, functional and structural brain abnormalities on multiple neuroimaging modalities and cognitive deficits are detectable in military Veterans exposed to mild TBIs. FDG-PET abnormalities and CSF tau abnormalities in deployed Veterans without TBI history suggest possible brain effects from environmental exposures. Longitudinal follow up studies of these Veterans would clarify blast mild TBI effects on risks for CTE and AD." (Peskind et al., 2014)

I find it necessary to comment in regards to the authors conclusions in the prior study. Their perception of 'environmental exposures' may or may not be correct but, what is unaccounted is in their research design is whether the combat Veterans had exposure to trauma within the context of their service involvement.

As discussed in the prior chapter, undiagnosed, untreated or incomplete resolution of PTSD symptoms have a clear association with the emergence of dementia.

The incidence of TBI among our returning Veterans is an important factor to ascertain. A 2016 study sought to screen all Veterans transiting through Landstuhl Regional Medical Center (LRMC). Each Veteran underwent TBI screening regardless of anatomic injury. The authors examined the incidence and various factors associated with positive screening. Their findings revealed that:

"Among 43,852 patients screened during the 5-year period, 6,594 were admitted, of whom, 6,590 received a complete TBI screen. Predominantly male (97.1%), the mean age was 26.7 ± 7.4 yrs. . . .Positively screened patients averaged 1.8 deployments, 69.5% experienced one or more blasts, 16.1% experienced one or more vehicular crashes, with 18.0% reporting a prior head injury.

"Of the 2,805 (42.6%) who screened positive for possible concussion, 2,393 (85.3%) were diagnosed with a concussion/TBI during their inpatient stay; the remaining 412 (14.7%) were identified by screening only. Of the screened positive patients, 1,953 (69.6%) reported 1 or more current concussion TBI-related symptoms; of those with symptom(s), 532 (27.2%) reported 5 or more.

"Early screening based on self-report identified a large number of patients admitted directly from the combat zone with possible deployment-related concussion and TBI symptoms. Such screening provides valuable information to guide decisions about early management and return to duty." (Connelly, Martin, Elterman, Orman, & Zonies, 2016)

Since the focus in this chapter is traumatic brain injury, I'd like to take a hop, skip and jump into a new world of red infrared-light that is promising change about which we previously could only dream. This world, of course, has its own language. Therefore, we will begin with some of the basic terminology upon which you may begin to build your understanding of this field.

Terms

Adenospine diphosphate (ADP): an important and numerous molecule in the body which is an essential ingredient for DNA. Its primary importance is in the storage and release of energy within the cell.

Both plants and animal forms of life utilize this compound. Plants use the energy from sunlight converting it into the formation of ATP. In contrast, animals take energy from glucose to build ATP from ADP.

Living cells cycle their supply of both compounds in about a minute. The conversion process from ATP to

ADP transfers energy to enable muscles to contract, receive and send ions that carry signals between neurons and release ATP to attract and bind with blood platelets to stop loss of blood and begin the healing process.

Adenosine triphosphate (ATP): refers to the "molecular unit of currency" of intracellular energy transfer which transports chemical energy within cells, including nerve cells, for metabolism. It is the high-energy molecule that stores the energy we need to do just about everything we do.

Amyloid plaque: sticky buildup which accumulates outside nerve cells, or neurons. Amyloid is a protein that is normally found throughout the body. For reasons, as yet unknown, in Alzheimer's Disease (AD) the protein divides improperly, creating a form called beta amyloid which is toxic to neurons in the brain. With the buildup of plaque, viscosity increases producing a 'stickiness' within blood cells. This is analogous to sludge building up in your car engine.

Central Executive Network (CET): refers to the conjoint function of brain areas working together as large-scale networks that involve cognitively challenging or demanding goal-directed tasks. "Resting-state functional magnetic resonance imaging (rsfMRI) studies have consistently shown that the CET and Salience Network, (below) negatively regulate activity in the Default Mode Network, (below) (Chand & Dhamala, 2016).

Cytochrome c oxidase (CCO): oxygen is an unstable molecule that is inclined to break apart and combine with other molecules in a process called oxidation. The instability of oxygen is used to power the processes of life. Food is oxidized in many slow steps, each designed to capture whatever useable energy is available.

The last step of the food oxidation process is controlled by Cytochrome c oxidase. By this time, all atoms have all been removed leaving a few electrons from the food molecules. Cytochrome c oxidase attaches these electrons to an oxygen molecule. A few hydrogen ions are added forming two water molecules.

Default Mode Network (DMN): Recent functional imaging studies have revealed . . . a distributed network of cortical regions that characterizes the resting state, or default mode, of the human brain. Among the brain regions implicated in this network, several . . . have also shown decreased metabolism early in the course of Alzheimer's disease (AD). We reasoned that default-mode network activity might therefore be abnormal in AD. The default-mode network appears to be closely involved with episodic memory processing." ("The Campaign for Modern Medicines,")

fMRI Scan Showing Regions of the Default Mode Network

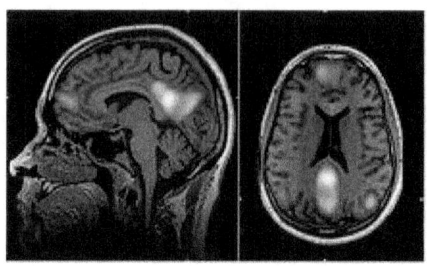

John Graner, Neuroimaging Department, National Intrepid Center of Excellence, Walter Reed National Military Medical Center

The default mode network, as shown above, is active when a person is not focused such as when the brain is in a state of wakeful rest-like daydreaming. It activates when the subject is planning for the future or remembering the past. This default model 'kicks-in' when the subject is not involved in a task. The DMN is negatively correlated with other brain networks that involve attentional focus.

Intranasal: lying within or administered by way of the nasal structures. Red infrared light provided for brief periods (25 minutes per day) has been found to clean and restore blood cells, reduce viscosity, lower blood pressure, increase cerebral blood flow, release melatonin, etc. The amount of blood traversing through the nasal passage has been found to be surprising high. Within the aforementioned time period, it is probable that all blood in the body has been exposed to irradiation exposure at least one time.

Irradiation: exposure to radiation from various sources. The term irradiation typically excludes exposure to non-ionizing radiation, such as infrared. Alternatively, the term is now being used with wavelengths longer than those of ordinary visible red light and shorter than those of microwaves.

Ischemia: a restriction in tissue blood supply causing shortage in the oxygen and glucose needed to keep tissue alive. The condition can be due a shortage of blood and oxygen to the heart muscle. It is usually caused by a narrowing or blockage of one or more of the coronary arteries that supplies blood to the heart muscle.

Laser: an acronym for light amplification by stimulated emission of radiation. A laser that produces light by itself is technically an optical oscillator rather than an optical amplifier as suggested by the acronym. It has been humorously noted that the acronym LOSER, for "light oscillation by stimulated emission of radiation", would have been more correct. The verb to lase is frequently used in the field, meaning "to produce laser light." When a laser is operating it is said to be "lasing."

A laser differs from other sources of light in that it emits light coherently thereby allowing a laser to be focused to a tight spot. Spatial coherence also allows a laser beam to stay narrow over great distances (collimation), enabling applications such as laser pointers. Lasers can also have high temporal coherence, which allows them to emit light with a very narrow spectrum, i.e., they can emit a single color of light. Temporal coherence can be used to produce pulses of light as short as a femtosecond.

Among their many applications, lasers are used in optical disk drives, laser printers, and barcode scanners; DNA sequencing instruments, fiber-optic and free-space optical communication; laser surgery and skin treatments; cutting and welding materials; military and law enforcement devices for marking targets and measuring range and speed; and laser lighting displays in entertainment.

Low Intensity Red and Near Infrared (NIR) Light: Infrared (IR): A radiant energy with longer wavelengths than visible light extending from the red edge of the visible spectrum from 700 nanometers to 1050 nanometers (nm). Light in this spectrum has been found to expedite the healing process by restoring the function of the respiratory chain. When this occurs, improved nerve functioning as well as increased blood circulation occurs through reduced viscosity and relaxation of the blood vessel walls.

Mitochondrion: an organelle found in large numbers in most cells, in which the biochemical processes of respiration and energy production occur. This is the energy factory of the cell. When cell channels are blocked due to Oxidative Stress (next) energy production is diminished. Light energy is selectively utilized by the cells in the body as needed. As the cells respond collectively, the effect becomes systemic. A negative feed-back loop is created in the body which triggers response in the system to initiate correction in the 'set point' back to a level of maximum wellness.

Oxidative Stress: An imbalance between the production of free radicals and the body's ability to detoxify harmful events through antioxidant neutralization. A free radical is an oxygen-containing molecule that has one or more unpaired electrons, making it highly reactive with other molecules.

Free radicals are able to interact chemically with cell components such as DNA, protein or lipids. The radicals have the ability to steal electrons in order to become stabilized. This can destabilize the cell component molecules, which triggers a large chain of free radical reactions.

Antioxidants are molecules in cells that prevent oxidative stress by contributing electrons to the free radicals without becoming destabilized themselves. An imbalance between oxidants and antioxidants is the underlying basis of oxidative stress which can lead to many pathophysiological body conditions.

Photobiomodulation (PBM): A technique utilizing exposure to light emitting diodes (LEDs) that stimulate cell functioning producing beneficial effects.
Damage to a cell through injury, the mitochondrion curls up thereby drastically reducing the production of ATP. In reaction, the rate of cell healing is drastically reduced or stops altogether. Cells exposed to infra-red light at specific frequencies cause the mitochondrion to spring back into producing increased levels of ADP.
 See Low Intensity Red and Near Infrared (NIR) Light: Infrared (IR).

Photon: An elementary particle that is an electromagnetic force carrier. It is the minimum form (quantum) of electromagnetic radiation, including light, and has characteristics of waves as well as particles. When an electron is excited by radiation, such as light, it receives and uses a photon, The electron will then decay from its excited state, emitting a photon. Undirected decay may be observed as luminescence. Directed decay may form a laser beam. Like other elementary particles, photons are best explained by quantum mechanics.

Respiration: While this term is often confused with the process of lung ventilation, respiration in fact refers to a set of metabolic reactions and processes that take place in the cells of organisms. The process converts biochemical energy from nutrients into adenosine tri-phosphate (ATP), and then releases waste products. The processes include aerobic respiration (glycolysis, oxidative decarboxylation of pyruvate, the citric acid cycle, and oxidative phosphorylation) and anaerobic respiration.

Salience Network (SN): Components of this network involve functions such as implementing and maintaining task sets associated with cognitive control, coordinating behavioral response, etc. The Salience Network plays a significant role in switching between the Default Mode and the central executive networks ("Salience network integrity predicts default mode network function after traumatic brain injury,")

Transcranial: passing through or performed through the skull. Various electromagnetic frequencies, including sound and light, pass through the skull and may affect underlying tissues at varying depths. Similarly, brain electromagnetic activity may be sensed near the surface of the skull (electroencephaolgraphy, magnetoencephalography).

Nanometer (nm): Infrared light is found within the electromagnetic spectrum. The varied wavelengths illustrated below are measured in terms of nanometers (nm) which is a metric measure equal to one billionth of a meter. The range of infrared light varies from 700 nm to 1050 nm.

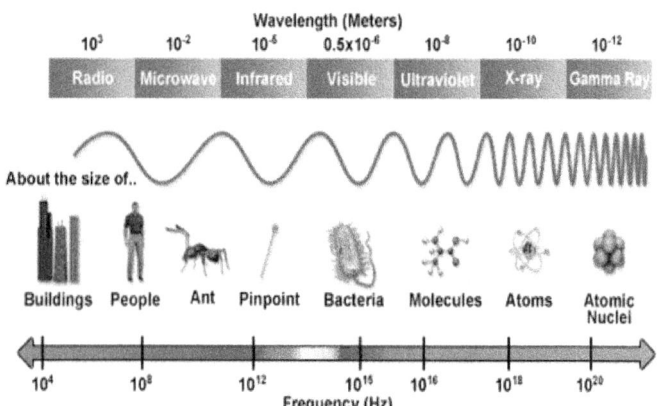

Electromagnetic Spectrum

Nodes or Hubs: A hub is part of a network with a larger number of links when compared with other nodes in the network. The number of links in a hub is much higher than for the biggest node in a random network. The existence of hubs is the biggest difference between random networks and scale-free networks. In random networks the degree k is comparable for every node and therefore it is not possible for hubs to emerge. In scale-free networks a few nodes (hubs) have a high degree of links while the other nodes have a small number of links.

At this point, we will shift to an exciting 2015 article by inventor, Lew Lim heralding the advent of an intranasal device that has shown efficacy in the treatment of traumatic brain injury as well as Alzheimer's disease. I have received permission from the author/inventor to fully utilize the material in his following paper ("Microsoft Word - Neuro inventor notes draft 1 Hil 2 - Neuro-inventor-notes.pdf,").

"For over a decade, transcranial PBM (Photo-biomodulation) have produced positive effects for laboratory animals and human subjects. Animal studies included acute traumatic brain injury (TBI), (Ando et al., 2011), (Wu et al., 2012a), Alzheimer's, (Purushothuman, Johnstone, Nandasena, Mitrofanis, & Stone, 2014) and stroke, (Detaboada et al., 2006) while human studies included TBI, (Naeser, Saltmarche, Krengel, Hamblin, & Knight, 2011), depression, (Schiffer et al., 2009), and stroke, (Zivin et al., 2009). Further, low level light energy has been found to be safe for humans in the stroke studies, without the side effects often associated with medications.

". . . There are sufficient data from transcranial PBM studies for me to develop applications with this modality. Unlike the possible adverse side effects of prescription medication, LLLT has no reported adverse effects or events that can be directly attributed to laser or light therapy. The high benefit to risk ratio of LLLT has been clearly demonstrated and should be better appreciated by medical professionals in the rehabilitation and physical medicine specialties.

". . . it is unlikely that photons from traditional transcranial positions on the head can reach the important primal regions of the brain that are located on the underside of the brain. In reality, these regions are much closer to the nasal areas than to the scalp. Amongst other functions, these regions govern memory, behaviour and emotions.

"In a nutshell, they determine the 'essence of the person' in everyone. The nuclei are located in these ventral areas (including the hippocampus, entorhinal cortex, and the ventral medial prefrontal cortex) and they form the important subdivisions of the key network of the brain called the Default Mode Network (DMN).

". . . light penetrates significantly more deeply into the brain from an intranasal position (in the nose) than from transcranial (on the head) locations, (Giuliani et al., 2009), it is logical that a light source located in the intranasal position is crucial if one is looking for a comprehensive PBM treatment of the brain.

". . . Unlike the transcranial method, photons from the nasal cavity area can be efficiently directed to the brain tissues, as there are no scalp and hair to act as barriers. . . This leads me to consider targeting only selected areas of the brain, which are the hubs of the key networks, primarily the Default Mode Network (DMN) and secondarily, the Salience Network (SN): Treat these busy and extensively connected hubs and the whole-brain would receive treatment.

"Default Mode Network (DMN). The DMN is of particular interest because it has been associated with Alzheimer's disease, autism, schizophrenia, depression, chronic pain and other neurologic diseases before 2010., (Buckner, Andrews-Hanna, & Schacter, 2008).

"Since the early discovery of the DMN, there have been many studies suggesting various nodes (or "hubs") where there are high levels of activity and connectivity. So, the health of the whole network is closely dependent on the health of these hubs. To simplify my quest for a set of hubs of the DMN to work with, I have chosen the hubs that are common denominators in the published studies such as ("The

Campaign for Modern Medicines,"), (Raichle et al., 2001), and (Greicius, Krasnow, Reiss, & Menon, 2003). Recently, Raichle further identified these regions as "subdivisions".

". . . The cells in the brain (neurons) are cells with mitochondria. To demonstrate neuronal response, Erlicher et. al., showed that weak light guides the direction that the leading edge of growth cones of a nerve cell would take. Therefore, when a beam of light is positioned in front of a specific area of a nerve's leading edge, the neuron moves towards this light and also grew in length in experiments that were repeatable experiments. In summary, nerve cells appear to thrive and grown in the presence of low energy light ("Guiding neuronal growth with light,")

"Further studies showed that cells in the presence of low energy light repair themselves. In addition, the neurites of neurons that were shortened by oxidative stress would re-elongate. The data suggest that red light irradiation protects the viability of cells and stimulates neurite outgrowth in cases of oxidative stress. (Giuliani et al., 2009), (Pitzschke et al., 2015).

". . . Light is an electromagnetic (EM) wave. A general principle about electromagnetic waves and penetration is that the longer the wavelength, the deeper the penetration. Radio waves are EM waves that are able to penetrate buildings easily, but the much shorter light waves are blocked by walls.

"Likewise, we would expect far infrared light, with its longer waves, to penetrate more deeply than red or near infrared (NIR) light with their short wavelengths. However, for tissues such as central nervous system (CNS) tissues, other components such as blood and water play significant roles in determining the depth of penetration. Researchers in the field of PBM have determined that the ideal wavelengths for CNS tissues are around 810 nm.

". . . A growing number of studies on CNS tissues and neurons using 808 nm or 810 nm have produced highly efficacious outcomes. One such study showed transcranial light therapy with an 808 nm laser diode attenuated amyloid plaque development in the transgenic mouse.

"This suggests possible efficacy of this therapeutic method using 810 nm for the all-important Alzheimer's disease in humans to penetrate soft tissues inside the nose. The treatment time is 20 minutes. Shorter treatment times require higher power but may create the undesirable thermal effect. Many healers believe the body requires 20 to 30 minutes to produce a healing response (Rojas & Gonzalez-Lima, 2013).

". . . In summary, the preferred set of parameters consists of an 810 nm LED light source, pulsing at 10 Hz with 50% duty cycle for 20 minutes. These parameters are the specifications for the Vielight

Neuro. . . when positioned in the nasal cavity, a large portion of the NIR light should theoretically reach the brain directly. . .

"Clinical studies show that visible red wavelengths are absorbed into the body's systems and utilized efficaciously. One of our science advisors, Dr. Timon Liu, observed many of these outcomes of intranasal light therapy on vascular diseases such as blood properties that affect hypertension and cholesterol levels." (Liu et al., 2012)

"The systems have been modulated into a negative feedback loop that restores the homeostasis states of its functions. (Xu, Liu, & Cheng, 2012).

"This suggests that although the visible red photons are not penetrating past blood and water, they are distributed throughout the body in some way and modulating its systems. Some of these results are expressed as measurable improvements in the factors that affect the hypertension and blood fats profile (including cholesterol levels).

"There is no available instrument to help confirm the biophysics of how the light particles are distributed throughout the body. Eastern Europe and some parts of Asia have offered intravenous blood irradiation therapy – by injecting low energy red light directly into the vein ("2_chapter_weber__final.pdf,".) The outcomes have been outstanding in many cases in a systemic manner. Later, our team as well as other researchers found that by increasing the power of an intranasal equivalent, the outcomes are very similar to the intravenous method."

****

A 2016 study by Wang, et. al., used broadband near-infrared spectroscopy (NIRS) to measure the LLLT-induced changes in CCO and hemoglobin concentrations in human forearms *in vivo*.

"Eleven healthy participants were administered with 1064-nm laser and placebo treatments on their right forearms. . . We found that LLLT induced significant increases of CCO concentration . . . and oxygenated hemoglobin concentration . . . on the treated site as the laser energy dose accumulated over time.

"A strong linear interplay . . . was observed for the first time during LLLT, indicating a hemodynamic response of oxygen supply and blood volume closely coupled to the up-regulation of CCO induced by photobiomodulation. These results demonstrate the tremendous potential of broadband NIRS as a non-invasive, *in vivo* means to study mechanisms of photobiomodulation and perform treatment evaluations of LLLT (Wang, Tian, Soni, Gonzalez-Lima, & Liu, 2016)."

Treatment results from the use of photobiomodulation (PBM) for traumatic brain injury as well as Alzheimer's Disease are quite impressive. Evidence of cognitive improvement has been forthcoming from a number of recent animal and human studies. I will first begin with some comments on the TBI/bTBI condition. Berman and Mills (2016) noted that:

Traumatic brain injury (TBI) affects about 1.9 million Americans every year. Blast traumatic brain injury (bTBI) has been called the signature injury in the Iraq and Afghanistan wars.

bTBI occurs without a direct blow to the head as seen in traditional TBI, but rather occurs as a result of overpressure from an explosion, such as a roadside bomb, that causes the vasculature of the brain to sheer leading to vascular insult (Berman & Mills, 2016)."

The historic beginning of low level laser therapy (LLLT), (photobiomodulation) occurred in the early 60's soon after the invention of the ruby laser in 1960, and the helium-neon (HeNe) laser in 1961. As discussed by Thor Laser:

"In 1967, Endre Mester, working at Semmelweis University in Budapest, Hungary, noticed that applying laser light to the backs of shaven mice could induce the shaved hair to grow back more quickly than in unshaved mice. He also demonstrated that the HeNe laser could stimulate wound healing in mice. Mester soon applied his findings to human patients, using lasers to treat patients with non-healing skin ulcers.

LLLT has now developed into a therapeutic procedure that is used in three main ways: to reduce inflammation, edema, and chronic joint disorders; to promote healing of wounds, deeper tissues, and nerves; and to treat neurological disorders and pain ("History of LLLT - THOR Laser")."

The terms "low level" and "cold laser" are also deserving of comment as discussed in the following 2012 article:

"LLLT involves exposing cells or tissue to low levels of red and near infrared (NIR) light, and is referred to as "low level" because of its use of light at energy densities that are low compared to other forms of laser therapy that are used for ablation, cutting, and thermally coagulating tissue. LLLT is also known as "cold laser" therapy as the power densities used are lower than those needed to produce heating of tissue.

It was originally believed that LLLT or photobiomodulation required the use of coherent laser light, but more recently, light emitting diodes

(LEDs) have been proposed as a cheaper alternative. A great deal of debate remains over whether the two light sources differ in their clinical effects (Chung et al., 2012)."

A 2016 article detailed critical information pertaining to deceased Veterans who had been exposed to blast injury. The authors noted that:

"Scientists have discovered a unique pattern of scarring in the brains of deceased service members who were exposed to blast injury that differs from those exposed to other types of head injury.

"Our findings revealed those with blast exposure showed a distinct and previously unseen pattern of scarring, which involved the portion of brain tissue immediately beneath the superficial lining of the cerebral cortex – the junction between the gray and white matter – and the vital structures that are adjacent to the cavities within the brain that are filled with cerebrospinal fluid.

"Those areas of the brain, damaged by blast, suggest that they may be correlated with the symptoms displayed by those who sustained a traumatic brain injury, or TBI," said Dr. Daniel Perl, study senior author and professor of Neuropathology at the Uniformed Services University of the Health Sciences. "This scarring pattern also suggests the brain has attempted to repair brain damage from a blast injury.

". . . Military members sustaining a TBI have often reported suffering from persistent post-concussive symptoms, which include a mixture of both neurologic and behavioral disturbances. These can include problems such as headaches, sleep disorders, difficulty concentrating, memory problems, depression and anxiety. Despite these prominent symptoms, conventional neuro-imaging for mild TBIs typically has not allowed providers to "see" brain abnormalities, leading this to be considered the "invisible wound," said Perl.

"This publication sheds some light, for the first time, into the nature of the persistent behavioral/ neurologic issues being reported in numerous service members who have been exposed to high explosives. It will certainly stimulate important further research and change how we think about these problems." (Shively et al., 2016)

One of the pioneers in the emerging field of photomedicine is Dr. Michael Hamblin who was trained initially as a synthetic organic chemist, later receiving his Ph.D. from Trent University in England. His research attention is now widely dispersed in the area of phototherapy for multiple diseases. Among his interests is low-level light therapy (LLLT) or photobiomodulation for wound healing, arthritis, traumatic brain injury, and psychiatric disorders:

> Applications of LLLT to healing and treatment of traumatic brain injury are being studied. Results from these studies have suggested that transcranial near-infrared (NIR) light may have wide applications to a diverse range of brain disorders, including stroke, neuro-degenerative diseases such as Alzheimer's and Parkinson's, psychiatric disorders such as depression, anxiety, PTSD, autism, and addiction." ("The Wellman Center for Photo-medicine: Faculty: Michael Hamblin PhD")

NASA has partnered with Quantum Devices Inc. to explore the use of Laser Therapy to negate the effects of muscle atrophy over extended periods of time in space. A NASA Spinoff posting noted:

"Specifically, Laser Therapy is the application of red light and near infrared radiation over injuries or lesions to stimulate healing and relieve pain without sensation or side effects. . . Many new applications for this treatment are being used and investigated including . . . nerve regeneration for spinal cord injuries and muscle atrophy for astronauts on long term space missions.

"The term adopted by NASA and U.S. military scientists is Photobiomodulation. Effective-ness of Laser Therapy depends on the color of the light (wavelength), intensity, and total energy delivered." ("LED Device Illuminates New Path to Healing")

A discussion of the nature of the cell and its component parts is forthcoming from the Pan Medica Healthcare Corporation web site with a mitochondrion diagram taken from a Wikimedia Commons illustration.

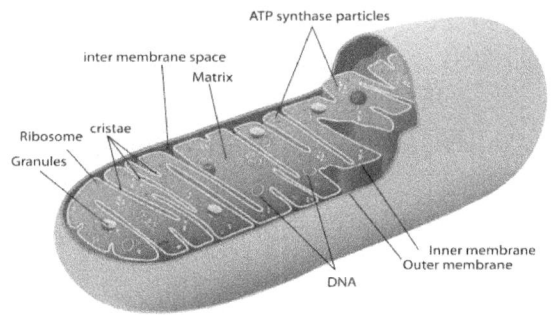

Mitochondrion

"A eukaryotic cell is any organism having as its fundamental structural unit a cell type that contains specialized organelles in the cytoplasm, a membrane-bound nucleus enclosing genetic material organized into chromosomes, and an elaborate system of division by mitosis or meiosis, characteristic of all life forms except bacteria, blue-green algae, and other primitive microorganisms." (Dictionary.com).

According to Pan Medica Healthcare Corporation:

"Every eukaryotic cell in an animal's body has one or many thousand cellular power plants called the mitochondrion. These mitochondria are responsible for providing most of the required ATP for cells. ATP is the chemical responsible for energy release within cells that drives a multitude of cellular and physiological functions including those directly related to injury repair and pain relief.

"When a cell is damaged through injury or trauma, the mitochondrion, figuratively speaking, curls up like a hedgehog. Once this happens, the production of ATP is drastically reduced, or even ceased. As a result, the rate of healing slows dramatically.

"Cells exposed to infrared light (Low Level Laser Therapy) at the right wavelength, causes the mitochondrion to spring into action almost immediately producing increased amounts of ATP together with signaling molecules such as nitric oxide and reactive oxygen species. Again, infrared light increases the production of ATP in damaged or resting mitochondria." ("Photo-biomodulation, Low Level Laser Therapy, Cold Laser Therapy)

We next explore animal models and studies pertaining to TBI, particularly those injuries produced from bTBI. This has been a challenging research area because of the need to develop an adequate injury-inducing model. According to Berman and Mills of Louisiana Tech:

"Experimental models for inducing a TBI suffer from two major disadvantages. Methods for inducing a TBI do not effectively model the mechanism by which TBI's and bTBI's induce structural and functional changes in the affected brain tissue. Secondly, most models are invasive with two injury sites, initial cranial opening and brain impact, and therefore do not easily lend themselves to further study of potential treatment modalities within the same experiment.

"We developed a model that better mimics the mechanism of a bTBI insult. We used an acoustic wave technology (a Storz-D-Actor device) to induce a consistent and repeatable non-invasive bTBI on Han-Wistar rats.

"The Rotarod test was used to monitor rat motor skills and the Morris Water Maze test was used to monitor memory. Controls received training but no exposure to the acoustic wave. Experimentally, one pulse of using four different acoustic wave pressures was studied: 0, 3.4, 4.2 and 5.0 bar (10 rats/group).

Each pulse was administered to each animal's left frontal cortex and rats were sacrificed after 11 days, brains process for histological analysis and stained with Cressyl violet for analysis.

"Results suggest that the Storz-D-Actor administered an effective and closed head bTBI that mimics bTBI blasts and caused a decrease in motor skills ability as well as a loss of memory.

"Histological analysis showed damage to outer cortex of the brain and necrotic neuronal cells. Our results suggest that the Storz-D-Actor can induce a damaging repeatable closed head bTBI that avoids the invasive procedure of a craniotomy and better mimics the mechanism of TBI (Berman & Mills, 2016)."

"A recent animal experiment by Xuan, Huang, & Hamblin, performed at Massachusetts General Hospital, did not use acoustic wave technology as described above. This investigation revealed that:

". . . Near-infrared laser photobiomodulation . . . delivered to the mouse daily for 3-days after a controlled cortical impact traumatic brain injury (TBI) gave a significant improvement in neurological/ cognitive function. However, the same parameters delivered 14X daily gave significantly less benefit.

"This biphasic dose response intrigued us, and we decided to follow the mice that received 3X or 14X laser treatments out to 56-days post-TBI. . . We conclude that an excessive number of laser-treatments delivered to mice can temporarily inhibit the process of brain repair stimulated by tPBM, but then the inhibitory effect ceases, and brain repair can resume." (Xuan, Huang, & Hamblin, 2016)

Wu et al., also working at Massachusetts General, used traditional means of establishing impact related TBI noted that:

"We tested LLLT in a mouse model of TBI produced by a controlled weight drop onto the skull. Mice received a single treatment with 660-nm, 732-nm, 810-nm or 980-nm laser (36 J/cm2) four-hours post-injury and were followed up by neurological performance testing for 4 weeks.

"Mice with moderate to severe TBI treated with 660-nm and 810-nm laser (but not 732-nm or 980-nm) had a significant improvement in neurological score over the course of the follow-up and histological examination of the brains at sacrifice revealed less lesion area compared to untreated controls." (Wu et al., 2012)

Other studies from the Hamblin laboratory have shown that:

"tPBM delivered to mice with TBI (Xuan et al., 2013), can upregulate expression of brain-derived neurotrophic factor (BDNF), a critically important molecule that can stimulate many aspects of brain function (Xuan, Agrawal, Huang, Gupta, & Hamblin, 2015). Moreover, neuroprogenitor cells (a type of stem cell) are increased in the hippocampus and subventricular zone.

"Neuroplasticity or synaptogenesis (formation of new connections between existing cortical neurons) are also increased by tPBM. Taken together, these observations suggest that tPBM can help the brain "to repair itself" after TBI, and this is likely to have implications for treatment of neurodegenerative and psychiatric disorders as well." (Xuan, Huang, Vatansever, Agrawal, & Hamblin, 2015)

Summary

In this chapter, the field of Photobiomodulation was separated out from other forms of emerging therapies. This was done for a number of reasons, foremost of which is the fact that Traumatic Brain Injury has become the signature injury of our current combat engagement in middle eastern lands. A second aspect that led me to include this information is that Photobiomodulation is yet another novel noninvasive treatment that seems to affect cell structure at its basic level with accumulating evidence of efficacy in the treatment of TBI.

Beyond the injuries incurred by Veterans through their exposure to IED's, close to 1.9 million Americans experience closed-head injuries yearly. Blunt force TBI and pressure induced bTBI were discussed and clarified. In a similar manner, "low level" and "cold laser" procedures that can reach deeper tissues and nerves through non-invasive means, with further research and inquiry, may offer hope to those who suffer with either form of TBI.

Research into the impact that blast exposure has on brain tissue has revealed a distinct pattern of scarring, which involves tissue beneath the superficial lining of the cerebral cortex. The damaged areas are believed to be correlated with symptoms evidenced in a traumatic brain injury. What is most encouraging in the post-mortem data is the suggestion that the brain attempts to repair damage from a blast in those who survived for a period after the damaging incident.

Discussion regarding the nature of the cell and the cellular power plant contained within it called the mitochondrion was provided. Note was made regarding the process of cell damage through injury or trauma, resulting in reduced production of ATP.

Exposure of cells to infrared light (Low Level Laser Therapy) at the right wavelength, causes the mitochondrion to spring into action almost immediately, producing increased amounts of ATP. I noted similarities to the 'tuning in' process used with RESET Therapy speculating that perhaps the mechanisms of action have some similarity at the cellular level.

Finally, the recent emergence of a research model that approximates the pressure wave injury forthcoming from bTBI offers us a greater understanding of how the injury occurs. Furthermore, it can also be utilized to assess the brain's plasticity as it attempts to repair itself as well as how it responds to varied treatment interventions.

Reference List:

2_chapter_weber__final.pdf. http://www .caferab basoglu.com/wp-content/uploads /2011/01/2_ chapter_weber__final.pdf

Ando, T., Xuan, W., Xu, T., Dai, T., Sharma, S. K., Kharkwal, G. B., ... Hamblin, M. R. (2011). Comparison of Therapeutic Effects between Pulsed and Continuous Wave 810-nm Wavelength Laser Irradiation for Traumatic Brain Injury in Mice. *PLoS ONE*, *6*(10). https://doi.org/10.1371/journal. pone.0026212

Berman, S., & Mills, D. (2016). Validation of an Acoustic Wave Induced Traumatic Brain Injury. *The FASEB Journal, 30*(1 Supplement), lb37-lb37.

Buckner, R. L., Andrews-Hanna, J. R., & Schacter, D. L. (2008). The brain's default network: anatomy, function, and relevance to disease. *Annals of the New York Academy of Sciences, 1124*, 1–38. https://doi.org/10.1196/annals.1440.011

Chand, G. B., & Dhamala, M. (2016). Interactions Among the Brain Default-Mode, Salience, and Central-Executive Networks During Perceptual Decision-Making of Moving Dots. *Brain Connectivity, 6*(3), 249–254. https://doi.org/10.1089/brain.2015.0379

Chung, H., Dai, T., Sharma, S. K., Huang, Y.-Y., Carroll, J. D., & Hamblin, M. R. (2012). The Nuts and Bolts of Low-level Laser (Light) Therapy. *Annals of Biomedical Engineering, 40*(2), 516–533. https://doi.org/10.1007/s10439-011-0454-7

Connelly, C., Martin, K., Elterman, J., Orman, J. A., & Zonies, D. (2016). Early Traumatic Brain Injury Screen in 6,594 Inpatient Combat Casualties. *Injury.* https://doi.org/10.1016/j.injury.2016.08.025

Detaboada, L., Ilic, S., Leichliter-Martha, S., Oron, U., Oron, A., & Streeter, J. (2006). Transcranial application of low-energy laser irradiation improves neurological deficits in rats following acute stroke. *Lasers in Surgery and Medicine, 38*(1), 70–73. https://doi.org/10.1002/lsm.20256

Giuliani, A., Lorenzini, L., Gallamini, M., Massella, A., Giardino, L., & Calzà, L. (2009). Low infra red laser light irradiation on cultured neural cells: effects on mitochondria and cell viability after oxidative stress. *BMC Complementary and Alternative Medicine, 9,* 8. https://doi.org/10.1186/1472-6882-9-8

Greicius, M. D., Krasnow, B., Reiss, A. L., & Menon, V. (2003). Functional connectivity in the resting brain: A network analysis of the default mode hypothesis. *Proceedings of the National Academy of Sciences of the United States of America, 100*(1), 253–258. https://doi.org/10.1073/pnas.0135058100

Guiding neuronal growth with light. http://www.pnas.org/content/99/25/16024

History of LLLT - THOR Laser. http://www.thorlaser.com/LLLT/history-of-LLLT.htm

Liu, T. C.-Y., Cheng, L., Su, W.-J., Zhang, Y.-W., Shi, Y., Liu, A.-H., … Qian, Z.-Y. (2012). Randomized, Double-Blind, and Placebo-Controlled Clinic Report of Intranasal Low-Intensity Laser Therapy on Vascular Diseases. *International Journal of Photoenergy, 2012,* e489713. https://doi.org/10.1155/2012/489713

Microsoft Word - Neuro inventor notes draft 1 Hil 2 - Neuro-inventor-notes.pdf. from http://www .t.emersonww.com/Neuro-inventor-notes.pdf

Naeser, M. A., Saltmarche, A., Krengel, M. H., Hamblin, M. R., & Knight, J. A. (2011). Improved Cognitive Function After Transcranial, Light-Emitting Diode Treatments in Chronic, Traumatic Brain Injury: Two Case Reports. *Photomedicine and Laser Surgery*, *29*(5), 351–358. https://doi.org/10.1089/pho.2010.2814

Okie, S. (2005). Traumatic Brain Injury in the War Zone. *New England Journal of Medicine*, *352*(20), 2043–2047. https://doi. org/10.1056/NEJMp058102

Peskind, E. R., Petrie, E. C., Pagulayan, K. F., Yarnykh, V., Cross, D. J., Richards, T., ... Minoshima, S. (2014). PERSISTENT BRAIN NEUROIMAGING AND NEURO-COGNITIVE ABNORMALITIES IN MILITARY VETERANS WHO EXPERIENCED BLAST MILD TRAUMATIC BRAIN INJURY IN IRAQ AND AFGHANISTAN. *Alzheimer's & Dementia*, *10*(4), P294. https://doi.org /10.1016/j.jalz.2014.04.487

Pitzschke, A., Lovisa, B., Seydoux, O., Zellweger, M., Pfleiderer, M., Tardy, Y., & Wagnières, G. (2015). Red and NIR light dosimetry in the human deep brain. *Physics in Medicine and*

Biology, *60*(7), 2921–2937. https://doi.org
/10.1088/0031-9155/60/7/2921

Purushothuman, S., Johnstone, D. M., Nandasena, C.,
Mitrofanis, J., & Stone, J. (2014).
Photobiomodula-tion with near infrared light
mitigates Alzheimer's disease-related
pathology in cerebral cortex – evidence from
two transgenic mouse models. *Alzheimer's
Research & Therapy*, *6*(1), 2. https://doi.
org/10.1186/alzrt232

Raichle, M. E., MacLeod, A. M., Snyder, A. Z.,
Powers, W. J., Gusnard, D. A., & Shulman,
G. L. (2001). A default mode of brain
function. *Proceedings of the National
Academy of Sciences of the United States of
America*, *98*(2), 676–682.

Rojas, J. C., & Gonzalez-Lima, F. (2013).
Neurological and psychological applications
of transcranial lasers and LEDs. *Biochemical
Pharmacology*, *86*(4), 447–457.
https://doi.org/10.1016/j.bcp.2013.06.012

Salience network integrity predicts default mode
network function after traumatic brain injury.
http://www.pnas.org/content/109/12/4690

Schiffer, F., Johnston, A. L., Ravichandran, C.,
Polcari, A., Teicher, M. H., Webb, R. H., &
Hamblin, M. R. (2009). Psychological
benefits 2 and 4 weeks after a single treatment
with near infrared light to the forehead: a pilot
study of 10 patients with major depression

and anxiety. *Behavioral and Brain Functions : BBF, 5,* 46. https://doi .org/10.1186/1744-9081-5-46

Shively, S. B., Horkayne-Szakaly, I., Jones, R. V., Kelly, J. P., Armstrong, R. C., & Perl, D. P. (2016). Characterisation of interface astroglial scarring in the human brain after blast exposure: a post-mortem case series. *The Lancet. Neurology, 15*(9), 944–953. https://doi.org/10.1016/S1474-4422(16)30057-6

The Campaign for Modern Medicines. https://modern medicines.com:443/item.php?id=alzheimers

Wang, X., Tian, F., Soni, S. S., Gonzalez-Lima, F., & Liu, H. (2016). Interplay between up-regulation of cytochrome-c-oxidase and hemoglobin oxygenation induced by near-infrared laser. *Scientific Reports, 6.* https://doi.org/10.1038/srep30540

Wu, Q., Xuan, W., Ando, T., Xu, T., Huang, L., Huang, Y.-Y., … Hamblin, M. R. (2012a). Low-Level Laser Therapy for Closed-Head Traumatic Brain Injury in Mice: Effect of Different Wavelengths. *Lasers in Surgery and Medicine, 44*(3), 218–226. https://doi.org /10.1002/lsm.22003

Wu, Q., Xuan, W., Ando, T., Xu, T., Huang, L., Huang, Y.-Y., … Hamblin, M. R. (2012b). Low-Level Laser Therapy for Closed-Head Traumatic Brain Injury in Mice: Effect of

Different Wavelengths. *Lasers in Surgery and Medicine*, *44*(3), 218–226. https://doi.org/10.1002/lsm.22003

Xu, Y.-Y., Liu, T. C.-Y., & Cheng, L. (2012). Photobiomodulation Process. *International Journal of Photoenergy*, *2012*, e374861. https://doi.org/10.1155/2012/374861

Xuan, W., Agrawal, T., Huang, L., Gupta, G. K., & Hamblin, M. R. (2015). Low-level laser therapy for traumatic brain injury in mice increases brain derived neurotrophic factor (BDNF) and synaptogenesis. *Journal of Biophotonics*, *8*(6), 502–511. https://doi.org/10.1002/jbio.201400069

Xuan, W., Huang, L., Vatansever, F., Agrawal, T., & Hamblin, M. R. (2015). Transcranial low-level laser therapy increases memory, learning, neuroprogenitor cells, BDNF and synaptogenesis in mice with traumatic brain injury (Vol. 9309, p. 93090C–93090C–10). https://doi.org/10.1117/12.2081022

Xuan, W., Vatansever, F., Huang, L., Wu, Q., Xuan, Y., Dai, T., … Hamblin, M. R. (2013). Transcranial Low-Level Laser Therapy Improves Neurological Performance in Traumatic Brain Injury in Mice: Effect of Treatment Repetition Regimen. *PLOS ONE*, *8*(1), e53454. https://doi.org/10.1371/journal.pone .0053454

Zivin, J. A., Albers, G. W., Bornstein, N., Chippendale, T., Dahlof, B., Devlin, T., … NeuroThera Effectiveness and Safety Trial-2 Investigators. (2009). Effectiveness and safety of transcranial laser therapy for acute ischemic stroke. *Stroke; a Journal of Cerebral Circulation, 40*(4), 1359–1364. https://doi.org/10.1161/ STROKEAHA. 109.547547

Chapter Three:

CHRONIC PAIN

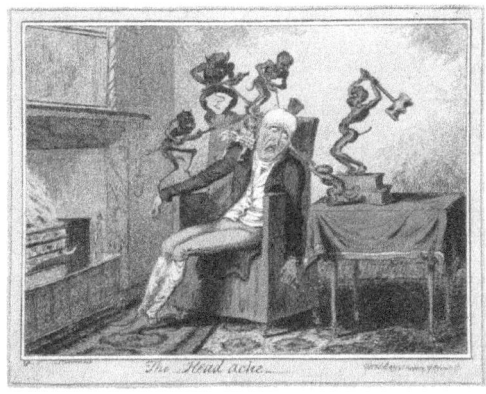

The Head ache

"Of pain you could wish only one thing:

that it should stop.

Nothing in the world was so bad as physical pain.

In the face of pain there are no heroes."

George Orwell, 1984

"Although locations and the names of conflicts may change, the physical and psychological toll on those who experience combat on the battlefield remains with them throughout a lifetime. Each theater claims its own signature wounds that emerge to punctuate that historical time. In our current conflicts, bTBI (blast induced Traumatic Brain Injury) and PTSD have taken positions of prominence with both often being referred to as the, 'unseen wound'." (Berman & Mills, 2016)

The focus of this chapter is on the topic of chronic pain. The directional flow of the discussion will take you to the beginning of battlefield medicine that truly began for the United States when it entered WW-I in 1917. From this historical perspective, I will provide you with my rationale for what I have come to call RESET-Pain Therapy.

I intentionally avoid discussion pertaining to the historical use of medication as it developed following WW-I as this would constitute a chapter within itself. (Paschall, 2016) Suffice it to say that medications for pain have been both a blessing as well as a curse for our Veteran and civilian populations in regards to the management of chronic pain. (Roux, Tang, & Drexler, 2016) In fact, a case study will be included describing the use of RESET-Pain as an alternative non-invasive approach for remediating intractable pain.

We begin with a historical excerpt extracted from Brenna K Pritchard's Master's Thesis (Pritchard, 2016) about the United States entrance into WW-I:

"When the United States entered the war in 1917, the army did not have an established medical corp. During the war, the army medical corps copied parts of the French and English medical system that had been in use for the past three years. This system arranged military medical staff in a practical manner.

Stretcher-bearers first came into contact with the wounded and moved them from trenches to waiting ambulances. The first aid treatment these medics gave often saved lives." (John Campbell, 1993)

****

Lieutenant Andrew Green wrote to friends in Raleigh praising the stretcher-bearers who carried him over one mile through enemy shell fire after he was wounded in the leg. Private Clarence C. Moore related that he "was a stretcher bearer in the Hindenburg Line for about half a day. We had to step on these dead soldiers to keep from going in the water and mud so deep and throwing the [wounded] off the stretcher" (John Campbell, 1993)

****

In the HBO hit series *Boardwalk Empire,* created by Terence Winter, we find ourselves visiting the Prohibition period of the 1920s and 1930s. One of the characters portrayed in the series is Richard Harrow, a former Army marksman who was disfigured in World War-I, wearing a tin mask over half of his face. ("Boardwalk Empire: Pictures, Videos, Breaking News,")

Richard typifies one of many disfigured Veterans who were maimed through their service in 'trench warfare.' Besides 'shell-shock', one of the lesser known signature wounds from that time was facial disfigurement, often caused by shrapnel. As the Veterans from this period pass away, the memories of the horror and pain they incurred are rapidly aging in the history books and old photographs.

Lest we forget their sacrifices, my way of honoring their service and sacrifice is to interweave aspects of their experiences throughout this chapter to remind us of the pain and horror they endured. We begin with a few paragraphs about the topic of facial disfigurement:

"The First World War saw a multitude of facial wounds, with veterans coming home with severe facial mutilation numbering in the thousands. These veterans have been somewhat overlooked in the historiography of medicine in World War I, and this work seeks to remedy that by examining every aspect of their lives, from the moment of the wound, to the aftermath of their return home.

"The medical professionals who treated these men gave a great deal of thought to the philosophy behind their work, and frequently voiced the opinion that their work was essential for the wellness of these men's psyches. This is because patients with facial wounds experienced a double trauma, resulting in both the loss of function and the loss of psychic identity.

"If surgeons were unsuccessful in covering over severe wounds, sculptors stepped in to take over for them, crafting fine tin masks for the men to wear until they themselves expired. The masks came to serve as a visual reminder of medicine's inability to cover the wounds of war.

"Finally, these men experienced unpleasant reactions upon returning home, because their wounds did not fit in with the way that Europeans preferred to memorialize the First World War. The personal accounts of soldiers and medical workers speak to this notion." (Pritchard, 2016)

Not only did these servicemen suffer unbelievable ongoing pain from the original injury but also, from the repeated surgeries they endured. To add further insult to their injury, they were perceived by those around them as being so grotesque that they were to be shunned and kept isolated in hospital wards.

Thus, a psychological insult was added to the chronic pain and physical component. In effect, the tin mask provided an altered persona permitting the Veteran to return to some semblance of civilian life when they returned home. The focus will now shift back to the issue of pain with segments of the tin mask story interwoven throughout the chapter.

There is no agreed upon definition for when acute pain becomes chronic. Some researchers suggest a transition time from an acute state to that of a chronic state within a 12-month period. Others believe that acute pain lasts less than 30 days. Other specialists suggest that chronic pain has no fixed duration but is to best defined as pain that extends beyond an expected period of healing.

The National Institute of Health (NIH) states that: "Chronic pain is often defined as any pain lasting more than 12 weeks. Whereas acute pain is a normal sensation that alerts us to possible injury, chronic pain is very different. Chronic pain persists—often for months or even longer." ("Low Back Pain Fact Sheet,") The Cleveland Clinic defines chronic pain as persisting despite the fact that the injury has healed.

> Pain signals remain active in the nervous system for weeks, months, or years. Physical effects include tense muscles, limited

mobility, a lack of energy, and changes in appetite. Emotional effects include depression, anger, anxiety, and fear of re-injury. Such a fear might hinder a person's ability to return to normal work or leisure activities." ("Safely Managing Chronic Pain | NIH MedlinePlus the Magazine,")

Chronic pain stems from varied circumstances including injury forthcoming from a motor vehicle accident, physical injury such as a fall, a traumatic event such as a physical or sexual assault or war related trauma or some type of disaster such as a home fire. Studies of the co-morbidity between PTSD and chronic pain reveal that about 15% to 35% of patients with chronic pain also have PTSD." ("Chronic Pain and PTSD,")

In sharp contrast, only about 2% of people who do not have chronic pain have PTSD. It is likely that the individual in pain may not realize that their pain and a past traumatic event are likely to be interconnected. It is estimated that approximately one in three persons suffer from some kind of chronic pain in their lifetimes with about 25% not able to engage in activities of daily living due to their condition." ("Chronic Pain and PTSD,")

****

"being wounded often caused a man to lose all sense of time and place. Half dazed, he lay or sat with gunfire all around, incapable of making effective sounds or gestures. The experience could be worsened considerably when one had received a head wound. In an essay written from the hospital in 1922. (Pritchard, 2016).

****

We (Lindenfeld & Bruursema) proposed that: pain sensitized circuits become locked in an overactive state, firing at higher frequency and coherence thereby producing the sensation of magnified pain. Once sensitized, these neural circuits can remain locked in this condition for years." ("Resetting the Fear Switch in PTSD,")

We further noted that neuromodulation is a process of stimulating positive change in sensitized nerves - essentially resetting the nervous system to a homeostatic state which brings about a reduction or elimination of the magnified sensation. We believe we can achieve positive results in many cases with safe, simple neuromodulation procedures.

A recent refinement of the above discussion has been provided. Before getting into the material aspect of the contribution, some definitions of terms are necessary. We begin with the term 'central sensitization' as noted in a web-page by Paul Ingraham that was updated on May 10, 2016. The author noted that:

"Pain itself often modifies the way the central nervous system works, so that a patient actually becomes more sensitive and gets *more pain* with *less provocation*. That sensitization is called "**central sensitization**" because it involves changes in the central nervous system (CNS) in particular — the brain and the spinal cord.

"Sensitized patients are not only more sensitive to things that should hurt, but also to ordinary touch and pressure as well, which obviously should *not* hurt. Their pain also "echoes," fading more slowly than in other people.

"In more serious cases, the extreme over-sensitivity is obvious. But in mild cases — which are probably quite common — patients cannot really be sure that pain is actually worse than it "should" be, because there is nothing to compare it to except their own memories of pain.

" . . . anything that hurts skin, muscles or organs — and it can be reliably detected with special equipment. The role of sensitization in several common diseases has been proven and well-documented, and may in particular be provoked by (common) muscle pain. It can also persist and worsen in the absence without apparent provocation.

Indeed, this neurological meltdown is such a consistent complication of other painful problems that some researchers now believe central sensitization is actually a major common denominator in most difficult pain problems. That is, it may be the nearly universal factor that puts the "chronic" in chronic pain, giving all such problems shared characteristics *regardless of how it got started* — not the *cause* of the pain, but perhaps the cause of its chronicity." (Central Sensitization in Chronic Pain,)

The next term that requires further clarification is Long-term potentiation (LTP). As provided in a long-term potentiation lesson:

"First discovered by Terje Lømo in 1966, long-term potentiation (LTP) is a long-lasting strengthening of synapses between nerve cells. Psychologists use LTP to explain long-term memories. That is, long-term memories are thought to be biologically based on LTP because humans cannot retain memories for the long term (the cells could not communicate with each other) unless connections between nerve cells are sufficiently strong for an extended period of time.

"LTP is also related to learning: without LTP, learning some skills might be difficult or impossible. In experimental psychology, researchers have induced LTP in mammals by repeatedly stimulating the synapses of nerve cells. Research on LTP has also focused on its relation to neurodegenerative diseases, especially Alzheimer's." (*Long-term Potentiation Lesson,*)

We are now ready to discuss a contribution by my colleagues John Garzione, PT, DPT and L. Richard Bruursema who note in a 2016 article that:

"Chronic pain is one of the most difficult problems to treat, especially when central sensitization (CS) has occurred. There are a number of articles in the literature that suggest that poorly managed pain leads to CS, which worsens with anxiety and lack of sleep.

"Long-term potentiation (LTP) causes a pain circuit to become hyper-aroused. It literally becomes "stuck" in a high-volume firing state. LTP maintains pain even after an injury heals, causing pain to become a chronic self-perpetuating illness." (Using Acoustical Stimulation to Enhance Neuroplasticity as an Adjunctive Treatment in Chronic Pain Management,)

****

To begin with, it must be explained that the sculptor does nothing whatever unless the surgeon has finished with the case. The wound must be radically healed. It is useless for the sculptor to tackle it if further shrinkages are going to alter its contours. When the healing is pronounced complete, the man can be turned over to the Masks for Facial Disfigurement expert, not before.

He enters the room, is seated in a chair, and very carefully scrutinized. He has been asked to supply, if possible, a portrait of himself as he was before he went to the Front.

Generally, he can do so. – that last photograph which the wife or sweetheart coaxed him to endure developes an unforeseen value! and this portrait guides the sculptor in some of the factors he must weigh in deciding what type of mask is best suited to the individual: later, too, the portrait will be of priceless help in the mask's finishing touches (Pritchard, 2016).

****

My colleague L. Richard Bruursema and co-author of ("Resetting the Fear Switch in PTSD,") conducted a personal capsaicin (cayenne-induced) pain experiment using the RESET-Pain protocol. The following is a review of his personal experience with hot chili paste.

"While eating some Indian food, I decided to add some very hot chili paste to bring up the heat level - just a little dollop in a larger amount of sauce. It got pretty hot. I started to get the typical burning tingle, heat, runny nose and watery eyes.

"Remembering that capsaicin had been used in pain studies, I decided to use myself as a subject. I took a large dollop of straight chili paste and placed it on my tongue. Sure enough, a very strong burning, tingle, heat and watery eyes and runny nose occurred. Instead of going for water, I held it in my mouth for 60 seconds, swallowed and then tuned in the RESET-Pain protocol and focused on the sensations in my mouth.

"Within 15 seconds or so, the burning began to abate on the tip of my tongue. The tingle remained but the 'pain' reduced to very little (estimate 75% to 80% reduction). But then I noticed the pain on my lips, so I switched my attention there.

"Within seconds, that pain began to fade but the pain on the tip of my tongue began to return. How interesting! So I switched attention from one area to the other for around 4-5 minutes. Each time I switched focus, the area of my attention experienced relief, but the other area began to feel 'painful' again. Over the course of 5 minutes both areas achieved around 80-90% relief without the customary water-drinking.

"I still felt a strong tingle and a sort of burning sensation - but it wasn't actually painful. It was a very different feeling as if the 'pain' aspect had been stripped out of the tingly-burn. Could this be amygdala deactivation? Since this sensory input is filtered through the amygdala, perhaps this is the experience of 'erasing' the amygdala threat-injury-pain content of the sensory experience?

"Day 2: While explaining this to my daughter, she asked if the effect was lasting, so I placed another fair sized dollop on my tongue and swished it around, bracing for the worst. Instead of the usual rush of - well, you know what it's like - I experienced a strong tingle, some sense of "heat" but NO pain. No discomfort to speak of at all. I could still enjoy the taste, and the warmth, but there was no 'reaction' like there usually is. But - this time I did notice a tangible, though lesser reaction far back on the tongue where I hadn't focused before.

"Day 3: Once again, a good dollop of chili paste on the tongue and held it there for at least 90 seconds and then swished it around. Once again, I found no discomfort, pain, runny nose or watery eyes. It still had a very strong tingling and sense of heat that I could taste fine - just no 'pain.' Interesting and unexpected: after I swallowed the paste (no water again) I started to feel a burning sensation and cramp-like pain deep in my esophagus, like heartburn. So the prophylactic effect was quite localized - to the area of my attention.

"My observations & theory on this: This experience duplicates the extraordinary specificity of the RESET-Pain protocol in other treatment sessions I have seen. For example, one woman had an all-over headache, but worse in the back of her head. She focused there and within a few minutes, the pain in the back was subsiding but not the pain in the front of her head.

"She had to re-focus her attention there, and then that pain also subsided. These results all point to the importance of attentional focusing to direct the effect of the treatment by more fully activating the target areas. It also duplicates the best-case results I've seen with the RESET-Pain protocol: not complete relief, but around 80-90% of the pain is eliminated.

"Speculating, I ask myself if the first big dose created a traumatic reaction in my amygdala, as though it triggered my limbic brain to perceive that it was really being burned and suffering an injury. I enacted a sympathetically aroused neural circuit specifically tied to capsaicin. Thereafter, each subsequent exposure triggered the reaction again. I truly didn't expect the lasting effect I have experienced."

Now you might ask why I would partner up with someone who would subject himself to such rigorous inquiry at his own expense. Some of you might not be old enough to remember the cartoon series called "Curious George." I identify with the cartoon-strip monkey's curiosity as does my colleague.

However, there's no way that you would get me to try that experiment. The above self-report is unquestionably subjective but now compare Richard's rather masochistic experience with the findings from a paper published in *Nature Neuroscience*. (Bonin & De Koninck, 2014)

"The researchers from the Faculty of Medicine at Université Laval and Institut universitaire en santé mentale de Québec (IUSMQ) were inspired by previous work on memory conducted some fifteen years ago by studies that revealed that when a memory is reactivated during recall, its neurochemical encoding is temporarily unlocked. Simultaneous administration of a drug that blocks neurochemical reconsolidation of the memory results in its erasure.

"The investigators wanted to see whether a similar mechanism was at play during neurochemical encoding of pain sensitization. To this end, they injected capsaicin in the foot of mice. Capsaicin, the pungent chemical in chili pepper, triggers a burning sensation.

"The procedure, which causes no physical damage, triggers pain hypersensitivity through a process of protein synthesis in the spinal cord. After capsaicin injections, the mechanical pressure at which mice would flinch was about a third of that in the normal situation.

"Three hours later, the researchers administered a second dose of capsaicin and, at the same time, a drug that blocks protein synthesis. The hypersensitivity then vanished rapidly. Within less than 2 hours, the pressure tolerated by the mice was back to 70% of normal.

"Yves De Koninck explains that 'when the protein synthesis inhibitor is administered alone, the hypersensitivity remains. The second injection of capsaicin is necessary to render the sensitivity to pain unstable and be able to interfere with its neurochemical reconsolidation. The challenge now will be to find protein synthesis inhibitors that are nontoxic and cause minimal side effects in humans.'"

Perhaps an alternative answer is the use of neuromodulation procedures to interfere with the reconsolidation process. If we could disrupt the chronic pain signal through non-invasive, non-chemical means, what a blessing that would be!

****

. . . the most interesting single development of the work here was the extensive use of cosmetic appliances to replace lost portions of the face, either temporarily, where surgical reconstruction of the lost organ was being planned, or permanently, when such reconstruction was considered impossible. As a result of much experiment among this line, a paste containing wax and gums, with colouring matter, has been invented, which is easily moulded, and reproduces most satisfactorily the appearance of normal flesh.

From this paste, noses, ears and lips are modeled and attached to the unfortunate mutilated person with surprisingly good effects. The method has a wide field of usefulness in rendering more tolerable the existence of these unfortunate people, and is worthy of employment in our own army.

A masking was considered successful when the patient could walk down a Parisian boulevard without being noticed. Earlier, after their multiple surgeries were complete but before they were fitted with masks, the men had gone on supervised forays into the city, accompanied by their nurses, only to find that onlookers gawked at them and sometimes even fainted. The men called this the Medusa effect.

The masks allowed them to regain some measure of the social visibility they had forfeited because of their ghastly wounds. (Pritchard, 2016)

****

Another colleague's response to chronic pain (we'll call him Barry) is included in order to elucidate his subjectively reported pain level reductions that attain levels of 80% through utilization of RESET-Pain protocols. As Barry is a trained professional with a focus on physiology, his findings are of particular interest. He reported that:

"I have a spinal cord injury at C-2 and I have diabetic poly-neuropathy that causes a synergistic pain effect that is heightened with neuropathy that is present in my hands, feet, legs, arms and shoulder as well as in my face. It is extremely painful and on a 10-point scale I'd put it typically at a 10. It's excruciating!

"I tried RESET-Pain with the initial protocol obtaining some relief, but not much. I kept trying the intervention and I'd get a little relief each time I tried it. One night, I tried it before I went to sleep and unintentionally fell asleep with the instrument left on. I slept through all of the night and woke up with my hands feeling 80% better. Now I use it prophylactically every several weeks or so when the pain reaches about a 6 or 7 level and the intervention then takes it down to a 2 level.

"With all of my years of physiology training, I haven't the slightest idea as to how the treatment causes pain reduction. The thing is an absolute mystery to me as I don't know how it works but I do know that it does work. The scientist in me says there's nothing I can put my teeth into about it that makes any sense. I am continually mystified.

"In the past, I've been real resistant to placebo intervention so I ruled that possibility out. The worst-case place of pain is in my hands because of the amount of nerve endings located there. Since this is the most excruciating target for me, this is where I focused with RESET.

"Interestingly, when I got reduction of pain in my hands, I also get reduction in my feet but not necessarily in my neck and face. I find that the pain tends to be site specific so I focused on the site-specific target that hurts the most and then I set the frequency dial and disruptor to a level that resonates with the site that hurts.

"I image my hand after closing my eyes. I set the frequency dial to where it resonates setting it uniquely each time I use it. I have developed an inner sense of what that resident resonant frequency is. I let it run until the pain begins to subside which can take from thirty minutes to an hour or two.

"Sometimes, I still have to sleep with it on. As discussed before, the effect seems to last for me for around two weeks which is better than any pain medications or anything else that I have been given. I've been using this probably over the course of seven months and I'm able to reduce my pain by 80% or so."

＊＊＊＊＊＊＊＊＊＊＊＊＊＊＊＊＊＊＊＊＊＊＊＊＊＊＊＊

The dead finally escaped the need to confront death; it was the living and especially the wounded who had to confront it. Disabled soldiers faced a desperate problem. Touched by grotesque death, they discovered to their horror that they had become the grotesque.

Robert Jay Lifton noted a similar experience among survivors of the atomic attack on Hiroshima. They had been touched by a death they felt was 'bizarre, unnatural, indecent, absurd.' Writes Lifton, 'After any such exposure, the survivor internalizes this grotesqueness as well as the deaths themselves, and feels it inseparable from his own body and mind. (Pritchard, 2016)

****

Another 'subjective' anecdote is offered as related to my own two and one half year condition of peripheral neuropathy triggered by my overuse of a large wet saw and the associated motor vibration to cut three-inch-wide ceramic tile kick plates for a condo I was rehabbing. This was further complicated by mild diabetes. First off, I will provide you with a review of the condition. (Peripheral Neuropathy Fact Sheet,)

"An estimated 20 million people in the United States have some form of peripheral neuropathy, a condition that develops as a result of damage to the peripheral nervous system — the vast communications network that transmits information between the central nervous system (the brain and spinal cord) and every other part of the body. (Neuropathy means nerve disease or damage.)

"Symptoms can range from numbness or tingling, to pricking sensations (paresthesia), or muscle weakness. Areas of the body may become abnormally sensitive leading to an exaggeratedly intense or distorted experience of touch." (allodynia)

I understand that this was a rather long-winded discourse on neuropathy however, given that 20 million Americans are experiencing this condition in some form or other and magnifying the number worldwide brings it to some astronomical figure, my RESET experience may offer yet another way to diminish suffering for some of those with this condition.

I would put my own circumstance in the mild category and therefore my reference to pain levels on the 0 to 10 scale is within this context. My symptoms include fairly frequent numbness or tingling, as well as pricking sensations (paresthesia), at times. Occasionally, my arms become sensitive to touch however, this has not attained a level of allodynia.

This issue causes me some difficulty with typing at times. I decided to try RESET-Pain following the results reported by Barry pertaining to his C-2 spinal cord injury and diabetic polyneuropathy. Additionally, I decided to begin an upper shoulder exercise regimen (I am notoriously lazy when it comes to working out) using machines available within my condo complex. In addition, I committed to a monthly deep tissue massage to address trigger points in my shoulders and neck region. The following report encompasses my personal RESET Therapy experience:

My first trial consisted of a 20-minute experience focusing on discomfort in my fingertips with the right extremities somewhat more severe than the left. I judged the level to be at a 6 reducing slightly to perhaps a 5 level at the completion of the intervention.

On the following day, after a good night's sleep, upon awakening the level was around a 3 in my fingertips. Amazing, the level in my feet was at a 0 with the complete absence of tingling of any kind present. Like Barry, my sole focus was my finger-tips so this seemed to be a revelation to me as well as a confirmation of Barry's findings.

Another week later, I retuned the Frequency and Disrupter setting, set the kitchen timer and laid down with my eyes closed sustaining focus on the delineated target. After 30 minutes the level was back down to a 1 with no tingling remaining in the feet.

The following day, the level of discomfort increased to around a 3 level in all extremities.

I decided to test Barry's surprise discovery that peripheral neuropathy pain requires more time than other targets due to the focus on nerve connections. I was able to get in an hour of treatment but was unable to fall asleep with the irritating sound on.

As an observer of myself during this experience, I noticed that my breathing was shallower then usual (diaphragmatic breathing comes naturally to me after 50 plus years of practice). I also experienced a slight sense of apprehension throughout the procedure. The sound continued to resonate with my target even when I became somewhat drowsy. Afterwards, only three fingers on my right hand had some tingling remaining at a level of 1 to 2.

My next intervention on the following day involved my actually being able to fall asleep for an hour and a half with the neuro-modulation sound on. Rather than using the prior setting, I fine-tuned the instrument to resonate with the remaining sensation in my right finger-tips. Upon awakening, I found that my left hand was basically normal as well as two fingers in my right hand. Three had slight sensations remaining that were barely noticeable.

My ability to type has significantly improved at this point. I theorized that varied frequencies are involved in nerves extending to the periphery and therefore, selectively tuning them in with each treatment is more advantageous than attempting to utilize the same frequency repeatedly.

This proved to be the case with my next intervention with the settings clearly different from the time before but still remaining at a low level, somewhere around the 1 setting. This went on for around an hour with my spouse clearly noting that I was snoring to my heart's content.

Thus, it seems that one can ultimately adjust to the sound and experience varied levels of sleep within the treatment process. At the completion of this session, all tingling was gone from the fingers on both hands. Some sensation remained in three fingers on the right hand but this was quite tolerable.

On the following morning, all tingling was absent in both hands with a 0-status obtained on the pain scale. I find these results to be quite amazing after a year and a half of discomfort. I continue to use this intervention as needed.

****

Strange to say the dawn of day brought me my misfortune... I had not been crawling outside many moments trying to get a view of ours and the German lines, when suddenly, I felt a smack on my face and a dull thud in my right shoulder. I was rendered speechless, and my arm hung at my side for many months afterwards. My friends looked at me in horror and did not expect me to live many moments.

They bandaged my wounds but they were unable to stop the flow of blood in my mouth which was nearly choking me. Then after a fresh telephone message had been sent which resulted in two bearers and a stretcher appearing about two o'clock next morning, I was carried out and a few hours later found myself in hospital. The doctors quickly operated and for a fortnight afterwards I was racked in torment. I have never been able to find out the name of that hospital. (Pritchard, 2016).

****

We now shift to my patient Hannelore (Chapter One), who had a colostomy in March of 2011 and developed complications two years later resulting in chronic wound problems. She ended up initially going to the emergency room at a local hospital with bleeding and had been treated at the hospital's wound center thereafter.

She noted having much difficulty with her wound recovery and consequently, we decided to focus on this specific target. Within this protocol, the patient adjusted the Frequency knob to resonate with her wound experience. She noted the following:

"It felt like stabbing. My mother said that I was raped and stabbed in the belly by the Russians. I've kind of pushed it aside all of my life. It started to weaken some. The sound is like pulsing and it became one with the pain in my belly. I was very anxious as I followed the sound. The anxiety got worse at first and then started to wane. I got an image of reaching for my mother. The pain has lessened from a level of 8 to a level of 3."

On her following visit a week later, the patient reported that she had a difficult week with her wound. She added that her pain has continued to be diminished perceiving that it was previously at a fairly constant 5 level and now remained at a 2.

"I'm still on edge with some nervousness going on. I woke up a couple of times like fighting someone off. In my early 30s, my pastor raped me. We worked on a church board together and I didn't like him that much. He had made suggestive comments to me before.

"I told my husband but he didn't do anything and we ended up going to another church. I was a victim again. I struggled against him."

RESET-Pain was again utilized with the patient asked to focus on this discomforting experience. Over the course of her 15-minute treatment, extensive trembling (muscle memory release) was noted that continued well into 10 minutes of her session lessening to a point of quieting over the last 5 minutes.

"It's amazing the feelings that come up - it becomes so real. At first the pain became more acute and then transitioned into the rape situation. I had lots of sadness. It was the Russian first and there was lots of pain and the scent of onion and garlic which made me feel nauseous and wanting to throw up.

"I have an aversion to them. Then it went to the pastor and I remembered more details. I had a sense of loss of my faith. I worked on it and got a better perspective. I would get flashbacks and things and it was a long journey for me. I want to be able to find something beautiful in things again and I believe that I can."

Before ending this discussion, I would be remiss to not discuss the type of injuries sustained in Iraq and other combat theatres through enemy utilization of IED's. Phantom limb pain is a form of neuropathic pain that is felt in an amputated part of the body from which the brain no longer receives signals.

It is estimated that nearly 82% of upper limb amputees and 54% of lower limb amputees encounter this difficulty. (Modirian, Shojaei, Soroush, & Masoumi, 2009) Vigorous vibration or electrical stimulation of the stump, or current from electrodes surgically implanted in the spinal cord all produce relief in some patients.

My summary perspective of current therapeutic treatments for pain is that the patient may generally expect limited reduction in discomfort with presently available interventions. At best, around a 30 to 40% reduction in patient discomfort is reported through varied interventions.

Results forthcoming from RESET-Pain appear to be much higher based on subjective reports of individuals using it (including myself) attaining levels of 80% or higher in a number of instances. While this chapter was initially intended to be limited to chronic pain associated with PTSD, I couldn't help but wander into ancillary medical applications such as peripheral neuropathy.

As noted earlier, "about 15% to 35% of patients with chronic pain also have PTSD. Memory circuits appear to be involved in sustaining the chronic pain effect thereby providing the possibility of RESET-Pain being able to alter this neuronal pattern. Subjective examples were provided as was formal research pertaining to changing pain reactivity by intervening in the reconsolidation process.

Summary

Addressing L. Richard Bruursema's personal experiment, Barry's unintended discovery and my application of his findings as well as Hannelore's alteration of her chronic pain condition all merge into a commonality that is clearly evident in the positive response to RESET-Pain.

As Richard speculates, the effects of RESET-Pain appear to be similar whether the selected target is emotionally traumatic or physically disturbing. If this proves to be the case, having the patient intentionally focused on the involved brain circuitry enables the reset of the emotional or physical aspects of the disturbance.

Further research is clearly necessary in regard to these findings as potential breakthroughs in pain management would dramatically alter the increasing use of highly addictive medications currently utilized as a mainstream approach to manage patient discomfort. The societal ramifications of such a study or series of studies, were they to produce results similar to the included subjective reports, would have enormous ramifications on the manner in which pain in our society is currently addressed.

Reference List:

Battaglia, A. A. (2016). *An Introduction to Pain and its relation to Nervous System Disorders.* John Wiley & Sons.

Berman, S., & Mills, D. (2016). Validation of an Acoustic Wave Induced Traumatic Brain Injury. *The FASEB Journal, 30*(1 Supplement), lb37-lb37.

Boardwalk Empire: Pictures, Videos, Breaking News. http://www.huffingtonpost .com/news/ boardwalk-empire/

Bonin, R. P., & De Koninck, Y. (2014). A spinal analog of memory reconsolidation enables reversal of hyperalgesia. *Nature Neuroscience, 17*(8), 1043–1045. https://doi.org/10.1038/nn.3758

Central Sensitization in Chronic Pain. https://www. painscience.com/articles/central-sensitization.php

Chronic Pain and PTSD: A Guide for Patients -
PTSD: National Center for PTSD.
http://www. ptsd.va.gov/public/problems
/pain-ptsd-guide-patients.asp

Jensen, T. S., & Finnerup, N. B. (2014). Allodynia
and hyperalgesia in neuropathic pain: clinical
manifestations and mechanisms. *The Lancet.
Neurology*, *13*(9), 924–935. https://doi.org
/10.1016/S1474-4422(14)70102-4

Long-term Potentiation Lesson. http://www
.chegg.com/homework-help/definitions/long-
term-potentiation-13

Low Back Pain Fact Sheet. http://www.ninds.nih.
gov/disorders/backpain/detail_backpain.htm

Modirian, E., Shojaei, H., Soroush, M. R., &
Masoumi, M. (2009). Phantom pain in
bilateral upper limb amputation. *Disability
and Rehabilitation*, *31*(22), 1878–1881.
https://doi.org /10.1080/09638280902810976

Paschall, S. M. (2016, May 5). *Chronic Pain and The
Prescription Opioid Overdose Epidemic:
Addressing Provider Attitudes and Concerns*
(Thesis). https:// utmb-ir.tdl.org/utmb-
ir/handle/2152.3/702

Peripheral Neuropathy Fact Sheet. http://www.ninds.
nih.gov/disorders/peripheralneuropathy/detail
_peripheralneuropathy.htm

Pritchard, B. K. (2016, July 26). Boys on Blue
    Benches: Disfigured Veterans of the First
    World War. http://etd.lsu.edu/
    docs/available/etd-07072016-124553/

Resetting the Fear Switch in PTSD: A Novel
    Treatment Using Acoustical Neuromodulation
    to Modify Memory Reconsolidation.
    https://www .academia.edu/12683048/
    Resetting_the_Fear_Switch_in_PTSD_A_No
    vel_Treatment_Using_Acoustical_Neuromod
    ulation_to_Modify_Memory_Reconsolidation

Roux, C. L., Tang, Y., & Drexler, K. (2016). Alcohol
    and Opioid Use Disorder in Older Adults:
    Neglected and Treatable Illnesses. *Current
    Psychiatry Reports*, *18*(9), 87. https://doi
    .org/10.1007/s11920-016-0718-x

Safely Managing Chronic Pain | NIH MedlinePlus
    the Magazine. https://medlineplus.gov/
    magazine/issues/spring11/articles/spring11pg
    4.html

Using Acoustical Stimulation to Enhance
    Neuroplasticity as an Adjunctive Treatment in
    Chronic Pain Management. https://www.
    academia .edu/27987707/Using _Acoustical
    _Stimulation_to_Enhance_Neuroplasticity_as
    _an_Adjunctive_Treatment_in_Chronic_Pain
    _Management

Chapter Four:

DEPRESSION

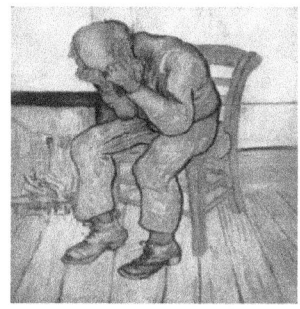

"Macbeth: How does your patient, doctor?

Doctor: Not so sick, my lord, as she is troubled with thick-coming fancies that keep her from rest.

Macbeth: Cure her of that! Canst thou not minister to a mind diseased, pluck from the memory a rooted sorrow, raze out the written troubles of the brain, and with some sweet oblivious antidote cleanse the stuffed bosom of that perilous stuff which weighs upon her heart.

Doctor: Therein the patient must minister to himself."

William Shakespeare, Macbeth

Historically, the treatment of PTSD has been both challenging and complex. Adding features of Major Depressive Disorder to the mix has led to a prevailing belief that patients with these concurring conditions are basically treatment resistant. The authors of a 2015 study suggest that:

> Prognosis is poor when the two disorders co-occur and treatment dropout is more common. People who respond to challenges and trauma exposures with negative affect may be particularly prone to developing both disorders and also to report childhood maltreatment. . . Finally, new treatment strategies that target the unique psychological and biological aspects of the comorbidity are needed." (Flory & Yehuda, 2015)

As expected, depression occurs quite frequently with PTSD, with prevalence estimates ranging from around 50% to 80%. Some researchers specialize in analyzing existing research studies that have focused on particular topics such as the relationship between PTSD and depression. (Rytwinski, Scur, Feeny, & Youngstrom, 2013) These authors concluded:

> An analysis of 57 peer-reviewed studies representing data on more than 6,600 civilians and service members indicates that about half

of those with post-traumatic stress disorder (PTSD) also suffer symptoms of depression.

As exemplified in the above, 'meta-analysis,' results indicate that 50% is a more appropriate estimate for a person to have both PTSD and depression symptoms simultaneously. With co-occurrence at these levels, it is not only necessary for a comprehensive treatment approach to be able to take this crucial factor into account but to remediate it as well. (Lenze, Blumberger, Karp, & Reynolds, 2015)

There are a number of types of depressive disorders; however, this discussion will focus on two primary types: major depression and persistent depressive disorder. In major depression, severe symptoms interfere with the ability to work, sleep, study, eat, or to enjoy life. An episode may occur on only one occasion in a person's lifetime; more often, the individual experiences several episodes. (Tylee, Gastpar, Lépine, & Mendlewicz, 1999)

In persistent depressive disorder, the person experiences a depressed mood that lasts at least 2 years. The individual may have episodes of major depression along with periods that are less severe but ongoing symptoms must last for at least two years to meet this diagnostic definition. (Kessler et al., 2003)

Treating the depression component is tricky because about 1/3 of people with depression don't respond to traditional treatment with anti-depression medication. This is referred to as "treatment-resistant depression" or "intractable depression." These are clinical descriptors for a depressive condition that doesn't respond to a minimum of a six-week trial of an antidepressant medication. (AHRQ Effective Health Care Program. (2010, June 15)

Because of the importance of the topic, we will begin by discussing the issue of suicide in those with the comorbid conditions of PTSD and depression. This will be followed with an overview of the impact that depression has societally, as well as economically. Additional discussion will ensue related to current treatment methodologies, discovery of a neuronal network linked to depression and a treatment intervention I've called RESET-Depression that offers an alternative way to address depression.

Psychotherapeutic interventions other than RESET Therapy will not be discussed comparatively within this book. The reader is referred to my second book, *Brain On Fire: A Therapist's Guide to Extinguishing the Flames of PTSD,* Chapter 6, Emerging Therapies, for information on this topic. I will also include case studies to provide examples of the effects that properly tuned-in neuromodulated sound has on the PTSD/Depression comorbid condition.

Our first inquiry will begin with a recent article pertaining to how well our Vietnam Veterans have adjusted over the decades upon their return to civilian life. The authors of this 2015 study inform us that:

> The long-term course of readjustment problems in military personnel has not been evaluated in a nationally representative sample. . . Approximately 271,000 Vietnam theater veterans have current full PTSD plus subthreshold war-zone PTSD, one-third of whom have current major depressive disorder, 40 or more years after the war. (Marmar et al., 2015)

When we put this information into context with the statistical likelihood of combat experienced Veterans developing dementia at twice the rate of their non-combat colleagues (Chapter One), we begin to see the emergence of an at-risk population that have remained silent and endured their internalized and hidden wounds of war for decades.

Another study (2012) sought to understand why more of our troops are killing themselves than are being lost in combat. These researchers compared Veterans who have killed the enemy in war to those who haven't.

"The United States military has lost more troops to suicide than to combat for the second year in a row and better understanding combat-related risk factors for suicide is critical. We examined the association of killing and suicide among war veterans after accounting for PTSD, depression, and substance use disorders.

"We utilized a cross-sectional, retrospective, nationally representative sample of Vietnam veterans from the National Vietnam Veterans Readjustment Study (NVVRS). Veterans who had higher killing experiences had twice the odds of suicidal ideation, compared to those with lower or no killing experiences . . . even after adjusting for demographic variables, PTSD, depression, substance use disorders, and adjusted combat exposure." (Maguen et al., 2012)

I described the Vietnam Veteran population as being an at-risk group that is clearly underserved in regards to the long-term consequences of their earlier trauma related experiences. Now let's take a look at the results of a 2014 inquiry related to those Veterans recently returning to civilian life in regards to how they are dealing with the comorbid conditions of PTSD and MDD.

> We examined the relationship of PTSD and depression, independently and in

combination, and rates of past-year suicidality in a representative sample of U.S. Army soldiers. . . Soldiers with both disorders (PTSD and MDD) were almost three times more likely to report suicidality within the past year than those with either diagnosis alone. Population attributable risk proportions for PTSD, depression, and both disorders together were 24%, 29%, and 45%, respectively." (Ramsawh et al., 2014)

The final article I will reference within this context is focused on Veterans utilization of an urgent care psychiatric clinic. One might interpret the findings from this 2015 article to suggest that our Veterans are finally seeking assistance for their psychiatric difficulties in a designated facility.

Unfortunately, a gloomier image may be just as likely. In this latter scenario, they seek emergency assistance as a last-ditch hope for some positive, life changing remedy. You, the reader, get to interpret and develop your view of what this data implies.

"Veterans attending an urgent care psychiatric clinic (n=473) completed a survey on suicidal ideation and other acute risk warning signs. More than half the sample (52%) reported suicidal ideation during the prior week. Of these, more than one-third (37%) had active ideation which included participants with a current suicide plan (27%) and those who had made preparations to carry out their plan (12%).

"Other warning signs were also highly prevalent, with the most common being: sleep disturbances (89%), intense anxiety (76%), intense agitation (75%), hopelessness (70%), and desperation (70%). Almost all participants (97%) endorsed at least one warning sign.

"Participants with depressive syndrome and/or who screened positive for post-traumatic stress disorder endorsed the largest number of warning signs. Those with both depressive syndrome and post-traumatic stress disorder were more likely to endorse intense affective states than those with either disorder alone.

"Our major findings are the strikingly high prevalence of past suicidal ideation, suicide attempts, current suicidal ideation and intense affective states in veterans attending an urgent care psychiatric clinic; and the strong associations between co-occurring post-traumatic stress disorder and depressive syndrome with intense affective states." (McClure et al., 2015)

I acknowledge that the issue of suicide might have been a chapter in and of itself. As there appears to be an increased likelihood that vulnerability is magnified with comorbid conditions, my plan is to comment on the issue where appropriate. Moving away from such an intense topic, let's explore the societal impact that depression has as a single entity disturbance. As discussed in a 2015 article:

"The economic burden of depression in the United States--including major depressive disorder (MDD), bipolar disorder, and dysthymia--was estimated at $83.1 billion in 2000. We update these findings using recent data, focusing on MDD alone and accounting for comorbid physical and psychiatric disorders.

"Using national survey (DSM-IV criteria) and administrative claims data (ICD-9 codes), we estimate the incremental economic burden of individuals with MDD as well as the share of these costs attributable to MDD, with attention to any changes that occurred between 2005 and 2010.

"The incremental economic burden of individuals with MDD increased by 21.5% (from $173.2 billion to $210.5 billion, inflation-adjusted dollars). The composition of these costs remained stable, with approximately 45% attributable to direct costs, 5% to suicide-related costs, and 50% to workplace costs. Only 38% of the total costs were due to MDD itself as opposed to comorbid conditions." (Greenberg, Fournier, Sisitsky, Pike, & Kessler, 2015)

"Pharmacological agents are one of several initial treatment modalities used for depression and one of the most frequently utilized classes of drugs are the selective serotonin reuptake inhibitors (SSRI). However, the rate of treatment response from baseline symptoms following first-line treatment with SSRI's is moderate, varying from 40 to 60 percent; remission rates vary from 30 to 45 percent." ("Treatment for Depression After Unsatisfactory Response to SSRIs - Executive Summary | AHRQ Effective Health Care Program,")

Thase, in commenting upon those who respond to antidepressant medication in an unsatisfactory way notes that:

> Persons with this type of response to medication are at greater risk for hospitalization, chemical abuse and suicide attempts. A strong genetic/biological component is often found within the context of this condition. (Thase, 2011)

Fortunately, recent scientific research has brought to light a cortical structure that is part of a neuronal circuit that endlessly recycles depressive ideation which produces a sense of constant hopelessness in the sufferer. Assuming that this information is accurate, then the quest for switching **off** the cortical signal that activates this neuronal network becomes of paramount importance.

Varied means of accomplishing this objective in cases of treatment resistant depression include non-invasive procedures such as ECT or RESET Therapy. Invasive procedures would include: ablative neurosurgical techniques, vagus nerve stimulation (VNS), and deep brain stimulation (DBS). A brief historical perspective will be provided to clarify differing perspectives pertaining to seemingly aggressive treatment interventions. As discussed in a 2015 articles the authors note that:

"Fossil records showing trephination in the Stone Age provide evidence that humans have sought to influence the mind through physical means since before the historical record. Attempts to treat psychiatric disease via neurosurgical means in the 20th century provided some intriguing initial results. However, the indiscriminate application of these treatments, lack of rigorous evaluation of the results, and the side effects of ablative, irreversible procedures resulted in a backlash against brain surgery for psychiatric disorders that continues to this day.

". . . Meanwhile, a significant percentage of patients remain refractory to multiple modes of treatment, and psychiatric disease remains the number one cause of disability in the world. These data, along with the safe and efficacious application of deep brain stimulation (DBS) for movement disorders, in principle a reversible process, is rekindling interest in the surgical treatment of psychiatric disorders with stimulation of deep brain sites involved in emotional and behavioral circuitry. (Cleary, Ozpinar, Raslan, & Ko, 2015).

"Deep brain stimulation of the major afferent bundle (i.e., stria medullaris thalami) of the lateral habenula has been used for treatment of depression where it is severe, protracted and therapy-resistant. (Juckel, Uhl, Padberg, Brüne, & Winter, 2009), (Sartorius et al., 2010)

". . . Even with Electroconvulsive Therapy (ECT), a significant fraction remains therapy refractory. For such cases, deep brain stimulation (DBS), is currently under investigation. . . Recent primate work implicated the LBh in controlling reward through the ventral tegmental area, imputing a "Circuit of Disappointment" . . .

"In summary, conversion evidence indicates over-activity in the LHb is present during the depressed state where it can drive changes in the mid-brain activity linked to depression. This proves that the LHb might prove to be a promising novel target for

DBS in cases of intractable major affective disorder. .
.

"Discussion: The DBS procedure resulted in a sustained full remission of depressive symptoms in a patient who was therapy resistant to all standard treatments for at least 9 years and suffered from severe major depressive disorder for 46 years." (Sartorius et al., 2010)

The above referenced case is quite impressive within the context of a case study. A broader perspective is to be found in a 2015 systematic review of deep brain stimulation through operative procedures for treatment resistant repression utilizing a Pubmed search. The researchers noted that:

"The study inclusion criteria consisted of: 1.) Diagnosis of Major Depressive Disorder, 2.) Well documented TRD involving failure of prior established pharmacological treatments, 3.) Controlled trials, uncontrolled observational studies and case series.) The measures of depressive symptomology pre and post treatment using a validated psychiatric scale to allow assessment of response.

"Overall, 10 studies were compiled and analyzed for this systematic review, with the number of participants in the study ranging from 4 to 30. 4 of the 6 studies showed 50% or more improvement in measures of clinical response in the subcallosal cingulate white matter /brodmann area 25 neuroanatomic regions.

"The ventral anterior internal capsule and ventral striatum sites of stimulation showed 71% and 23% clinical response rates in 2 studies. The nucleus accumbens elicited a 45% clinical response rate. Finally, the supero-lateral branch of the medial forebrain bundle (bilaterally) resulted in 86% clinical response rate in 1 study." (Aiyer & Joffe, 2015)

A concluding note on this topic follows:

> . . . DBS does involve a neurosurgical procedure. Electrodes connected to a subcutaneous implantable pulse generator (IPG), which controls stimulation and provides power, are stereotactically implanted into a specific brain region. In general, the procedure is well tolerated, with the most common adverse events directly associated with the surgical procedure or device failure: perioperative headache, infection, hemorrhage, seizure, and lead fracture. (Ryder & Holtzheimer, 2016)

Now I don't know about you folks, but I don't believe that I'd look kindly about someone drilling a hole or two in my head, putting rods in the holes and then hooking me up to a wire or two. I'm guessing that I'd seek to explore a less rigorous, non-invasive procedure with minimal side-effects. Alternatively, if I were suffering from depression for 46 years, I mightn't be in a position to make such a decision and would probably grasp at anything that might offer hope.

A shift is in order moving us from desperation to hope by inquiring about a principal site associated with depression referred to as the Lateral Habenula (LHb). This organ anatomically involves the stalk that connects the pineal gland to the rest of the brain. Input to the LHb is received from areas of the brain that are involved in reward as well as emotional processing, including the basal ganglia.

The LHb circuit itself is associated with both excitatory and inhibitory neurons. Although this sounds counter-intuitive, too much excitement in this circuit is associated with depression, while diminished activity is linked with sensations ranging from contentment to joy. As reported in a 2014 article pertaining to this topic:

> The brain reward circuit has a central role in reinforcing behaviors that are rewarding and preventing behaviors that lead to punishment.

Recent work has shown that the lateral habenula is an important part of the reward circuit by providing 'negative value' signals to the dopaminergic and serotonergic systems. (Proulx, Hikosaka, & Malinow, 2014)

The Lateral Habenula (LHb) circuit is quite complex and very different from that of the limbic system model. I have been using RESET-Depression or, as I have come to call it, the **Disappointment, Despair, Depression** or **3-D's** circuit of the brain when discussing the depressive recycling effect with patients.

RESET-Depression is showing amazing results in altering deep-seated depression in my patients. It is now a standard part of my PTSD intervention after the traumatic memories have been RESET. I'll provide you with information pertaining to this brain area, its connections and circuitry, treatment interventions designed to alter the circuitry and then suggest how the RESET-Depression protocol likely affects it.

A 2014 study focused on an area of the brain that specializes in predicting rewards by showing increases in activity in response to enjoyable things such as food, sex or drugs.

"Activity in these areas informs us when things are about to get good. But for every high there is a low. The Lateral Habenula is thought to play a role in how we process negative events: Getting a lemon on the slot machine again or the empty inbox on your dating site. . .

"Studies in monkeys and other animals have shown that increased activity in the Habenula is linked to depressive behaviors, and treatment with antidepressants decreases this activity." (Hsu et al., 2014)

To date, no formal fMRI inquiry has been done that examines the effects of RESET-Depression on the LHb circuitry. The same can be said for the RESET-Anxiety model. This work is clearly indicated given the results cited in numerous case studies. However, I will speculate that with PTSD we seek to turn the cortical circuitry off to assist the patient to revert back to a growth mode.

With depression, our intent is to diminish the LHb contribution thereby energizing the suppressed pleasure centers. In this sense, visualize a scale that is balanced rather than primarily tipped in one direction.

As a general rule of thumb, I focus first on trauma-related issue till the circuit is cleared. Generally, the proof for this is conveyed in the patient's statement of sleeping soundly (perhaps for the first time in years) and being free of the intrusive nightmares that had so prevailed.

When this goal has been accomplished (it can occur relatively quickly in uncomplicated cases), I will next explore disappointments, despair and depression issues. As you will read in the chapter about Survivor's Guilt, this issue may emerge at this point in time as well.

Practically speaking, the 3-D's or RESET-Depression clinical intervention proceeds more slowly than does the PTSD/trauma intervention. There are exceptions, but my clinical experience suggests that the therapist should expect gradual ongoing therapeutic breakthroughs that are accompanied by emerging levels of insight on the part of the patient.

I believe that this is part of the normalization process that occurs with a transformative revitalization of the now reset PTSD Neuronal Network. In particular, as the pre-frontal lobes are freed from the effects of trauma, insight emerges.

I always forewarn my patient that he/she will likely experience fleeting moments of pleasure that emerge from the brains pleasure centers. The cortical reward system consists of brain structures that are associated with positive reinforcement that consists of two parts. The first is the desire component and the second, the pleasure component. These aspects tend to emerge as the LHb influence is diminished.

I will also prepare my patient for the potential outbreak of cathartic release that may include the "shake, rattle and roll" phenomenon that I've seen when RESET-Therapy is successful in putting the brakes on the LHb circuit. By "shake, rattle and roll," I mean that the muscular system may also simultaneously release stored muscle tension locked in the memory circuit that is caused by a pent up emotional charge. As asked by the noted author, Dr. Peter Levine:

"So what is the therapist to *do* with human beings hurt and beaten down by past trauma? It is to help people listen to the unspoken voice of their own bodies and to enable them to feel their "survival emotions" of rage and terror without being overwhelmed by these powerful states. . . Trauma is caused when we are unable to release blocked energies, to move fully through the physical/emotional reactions to hurtful experiences. Trauma is not what happens to us, but what we hold inside in the absence of an empathic listener.

"The salvation, then, is to be found in the body. "Most people," Levine notes, "think of trauma as a 'mental' problem, even as a 'brain disorder.' However, trauma is something that happens in the body." . . . Hence," talking cures" that engage the intellect or even the emotions do not reach deep enough.

"Potentially traumatic situations are ones that induce states of high physiological arousal but without the freedom of the affected individual to get past these states: danger without the possibility of fight or flight, and afterward, without the opportunity to "shake it off," as a wild animal would following an encounter with a predator.

"What ethnologists call *tonic immobility* - the paralysis and emotional shutdown that characterizes the universal experience of helplessness in the face of mortal danger – comes to dominate the person's life and functioning. We are "scared stiff." In human beings, unlike in animals, the *state* of temporary freezing becomes a long-term *trait*. The survivor, Peter Levine points out, remains "stuck in a kind of limbo not fully reengaging in life." (Levine, 2010)

At this point, I can only speculate that there is a connection between the neural circuitry associated with the LHb and that associated with the above described muscular release.

Profuse crying that may come in waves is another release that will often occur. With each ensuing treatment, it is as if layer after layer peels off with a lightening of spirit that accompanies the process. Typically, even after intense crying, the patient will note a positive sensation upon the completion of the treatment session.

It is critically important that the patient be forewarned of this release possibility before the 3-D's treatment intervention begins in order to avoid a weakening of trust in the therapist. To do so afterwards invites skepticism and the high probability that the patient will halt the treatment process due to immense fear and uncertainty of what is yet to come.

Throughout the treatment experience, I advise my patient to remain skeptical until otherwise self-convinced. I describe the peeling away process related to the layering of depressive material and the consequent lightening of internal pressure forthcoming from the release of emotional poison contained within.

I explain that our objective is to deactivate the LHb neuronal network thereby energizing suppressed circuitry associated with pleasure and happiness. For those who are confused with this explanation, I use a seesaw analogy noting that we are gradually tipping the seesaw to a more positive position.

Let us assume that the patient has been fully educated regarding matters pertaining to reconsolidation, resonance, the BAUD, etc. I proceed to instruct the individual in 'tuning in' the 3-D circuit. Specifically, the Volume Knobs on the BAUD are set by the patient with closed eyes so that the focus is directed to the sound level rather than the numbers on the knobs. Once set, the volume remains in the same position for all protocols.

The next step involves the Frequency Knob which is adjusted by the therapist to resonate, via patient feedback, with selected targets. Typically, this begins with mildly disturbing targets such as that of disappointment of some kind. I would suggest that the selected target be in the 4 to 6 range on the 0 to 10 scale with 10 representing the most disturbing level. I have found that when the patient begins with a highly charged emotional target, it is likely to 'kick-off' a strong emotional release (cathartic) for which the patient is not fully prepared.

Next, the Disrupter Knob is also set by the therapist, via patient feedback, to weaken the strength of the forthcoming disappointment material. The patient is instructed to "tune in" to the full spectrum experience of disappointment initially, but then to let the inner mind lead the way to bring up whatever target it chooses. A number of my patients expected a particular scenario to emerge at a subconscious level and were utterly amazed at what did actually present.

Frequently, the response was something to the effect that, "I haven't thought of that in years!" I believe that by rebalancing the LHb to a more neutral position, connectivity is strengthened to the prefrontal lobe enabling a freer flow of ideation to the conscious mind. A brief 3-D case study will provide you with an understanding of why I am so enthused about RESET-Depression.

"I was born November 13, 1971 as Sean R. and never got to meet the man who was my biological father because my mother said that he was the leader of a motorcycle gang. My mother thought that would not be a good life for her children to live.

"Around the time, I was getting ready to start school, my two uncles were in the headlines of the newspaper because they had abducted, raped, murdered and burned two young teenage girls. My mother thought it would be wise to change her last name so her husband adopted me and my brother.

"Now I am known as Sean O. I never knew the man who gave us our name since we were so young. Unfortunately, my mother married a man who was very abusive to me and my brother. My mother divorced him because of this. I lived with my grandparents up to the age of 8 and my grandfather was the only father I had ever known.

"During my youth, my brother was very physically abusive to me. I felt like he got enjoyment out of beating me up. There's 15 months' age difference between me and my older brother. He would beat me up daily and sometimes for no good reason.

"My brother wouldn't leave any physical marks for anyone to see and he'd threaten me if I had told on him. My mother never knew what my brother was doing to me. She was a single mom working multiple jobs. The abuse which included both physical and mental went on for 14 years. Not once in all the 14 years did I ever hit my brother back because he was my brother and I didn't think I should hurt him. I felt if I let it go, the rage inside me would have probably killed him.

"On my third and final visit with Doctor Lindenfeld, he asked me how things were going and I told him that I only had one episode of night sweats. At first, I didn't think that there was anything wrong but he suggested that we do a slightly different kind of treatment with the sound that he called a "disappointment /depression protocol".

"I thought long and hard and the only thing I could come up with that was still bothering me was my brother. I mentally reviewed the timeline of my life thinking about my youth and my relationship with my brother while listening to the sound.

"I couldn't believe it but all of a sudden, I felt like a tidal wave of emotion came over me and I burst into continuous tears and sobbing. All I could say during that explosion of emotions was, he was my brother and he was supposed to protect me. After that release, I felt like the weight of the world had come off my shoulders.

"In retrospect, my brother and I dealt differently with not knowing our father. I couldn't miss someone I never knew. My brother idealized him and couldn't seem to get away from the loss. I grew up never getting in trouble and always trying to do what was right.

"My brother is presently serving 12 years in prison for attempted murder. He's been in and out of prison since he was 18 and he is presently 44 years old. I haven't spoken to him in over 25 years. I've come to forgive him and feel sorry for him.

"After that last RESET Therapy session, I felt exhausted. I felt like every ounce of energy had been sucked from my body. I drove home, talked to my wife a little bit and went to bed because I was so tired. The next morning, I awoke with a profound sense of being a new man.

"Since the last treatment, I've come to enjoy life, no more cold-sweats, sleepless nights or being an ass-hole. The three things that I'm so happy about are that I'm smiling again, I'm laughing again and I found joy in my life."

Next, we'll compare the protocol I've named the 3-D's (disappointment, despair, depression) with other current interventions for the 1/3 of patients who do not respond to anti-depressant medications. As an aside, the mechanisms of many of these treatments remain unknown such as those of Electroconvulsive Therapy (ECT).

The current therapeutic options for treatment-resistant depression are problematic in several ways. First, there is the cost factor, since many of these options aren't covered by the insurance industry. Second, there is the risk factor related to doing more harm than good to the individual. Finally, there are issues with the availability and frequency of these interventions.

Electroconvulsive Therapy (ECT) still remains controversial because it consists of providing electrical currents to targeted areas of the brain to induce a seizure effect. This certainly seems to be counterintuitive; however, the procedure remains in use, having diminished from its broad usage in the 1960's for a wide variety of conditions.

Selected excerpts from a 2013 article are provided here related to features common to ECT as well as RESET Therapy. Certainly, elements of stress are a common feature with both procedures. For example, each approach speculates about the presence of impaired feedback regulation controlled by the frontotemporal structures. (Canu et al., 2015)

"EEG data indicate that activation and deactivation of under-aroused and hyper-aroused neuronal networks are triggered by both procedures. Though the mechanism of action of the neuromodulation effect has been alluded to ("PTSD,"), the exacts mechanisms by which ECT acts still remain a mystery.

"More than 70 years after its inception, no consensus has been reached on the mode of action of electroconvulsive treatment (ECT). . . altered structure and functioning is seen in the hypothalamic-pituitary-adrenal (HPA) stress axis, including hypersensitivity to stressors, chronically elevated levels of stress hormones and impaired feedback regulation by frontotemporal structures. . . etiologically, the HPA axis alterations are consistent with stress-exposure as a significant factor in severe depression.

"Stress activates the mesocorticolimbic dopamine system as well as the HPA axis. . . We hypothesize that anti-depressive effects of ECT reflect the impact of the intervention upon these systems that are altered in depression.

". . . The impact of ECT upon frontotemporal activity has been investigated by both electroencephalography (EEG) and brain imaging techniques, in recent decades mainly by positron emission tomography (PET) and single photon emission computed tomography (SPECT), but also by functional magnetic resonance imaging (fMRI).

"We focus on studies that reported changes in brain activity level from before to after ECT as evidenced by increases (which we term activation) and decreases (deactivation) in the EEG power spectrum and cerebral blood flow." (Fosse & Read, 2013)

ECT currently remains a fallback option for those experiencing severe depression. The treatment itself extends over a 10 to 15-minute period after the patient is provided with anesthesia. Typically, two to three sessions are provided per week for two to four weeks.

Within the context of his discussion, Dr. Chittaranjan Andrade suggested that a clinician may explain ECT to the patient as follows:

"Delivery of a small but adequate dose of electricity to the brain results in the elicitation of seizure activity in the brain; higher electrical doses elicit a better quality of seizure. The seizure releases a large number of signaling chemicals that, in turn, produce changes on the surface and then within nerve and glial cells in target areas of the brain such as the hippocampus, amygdala, and prefrontal cortex.

"Genes in these cells are activated or suppressed, which in turn leads to change in the number, activity, and connectivity of these cells. Increased number and connectivity of cells in the hippocampus and prefrontal cortex probably improve thinking and coping abilities, whereas decreased number and connectivity of cells in the amygdala reduce negative emotions attached to unpleasant memories; both effects can be expected to be therapeutic in depressed patients. The time course of recovery from depression seems to parallel the time course of occurrence of these cellular changes." (Andrade, 2014)

Once again, the brain regions referenced by Dr. Andrade such as the amygdala and pre-frontal cortex are in the same cortical brain regions as those involved with PTSD and other forms of anxiety as discussed previously with respect to the mechanisms of action of RESET Therapy.

We might therefore argue that auditory stimulation, also an invasive procedure when compared to ECT because it uses an external stimulus to modify activity in central neuronal networks, is a more humane and benign procedure. The differences between the two treatments lie in such areas as stimulus-responses specificity, stimulus strength, the severity of side effects, and the quality of the treatment outcome, with RESET being superior to ECT in each area.

A benign approach avoids the multiple side effects of ECT that can include adverse reaction to anesthetic agents and neuromuscular blocking agents, alterations in blood pressure, cardiovascular complications, death, dental and oral trauma, pain and discomfort, physical trauma, prolonged seizures, pulmonary complications, skin burns, and stroke, cognitive and memory dysfunction, and device malfunction.

Furthermore, is it possible that a number of non-responders to anti-depressant medication may have experienced trauma that caused the depression in the first place? As described in the following article, the patient was traumatized by rape and was unable to verbalize her experience.

As you will read below, her treating doctors missed this vital aspect of her condition and proceeded to treat her based on erroneous information. This is the first of two case examples that I present here to illustrate differing perspectives on the use of ECT.

"At age 16 I was raped. I suffered severe post-traumatic shock and was taken to a psych ward. I was in a non-verbal state and the psychiatrist upon admission misdiagnosed my condition as "catatonic schizophrenia." After only four days of observation I was started on a course of 10 shock treatments - which in and of themselves were as traumatizing as the rape.

"When I awoke after each "treatment" I felt completely broken, like a walking zombie. I experienced ECT as invasive, cruel and terrifying. Today, 25 years later, my memory and abilities to comprehend and learn are still greatly disabled. I have permanent brain damage from this form of 'therapy.'

"Shock treatment was the most horrific experience in my life. If you think you're losing your mind - have ECT, and for certain you will." (Purse,)

In contrast, the following story was provided about John Wattie, age sixty-four who reported that his breakdown in the late 1990's was triggered by the collapse of his marriage and stress at work.

> We had a nice house and a nice lifestyle, but it was all just crumbling away. My depression was starting to overwhelm me. I lost control, I became violent. I liken the feeling to being in a hole, a hole I could not get out of despite courses of pills and talking therapies. Before ECT, I was the walking dead. I had no interest in life, I just wanted to disappear. After ECT, I felt like there was a way out of it. I felt dramatically better ("Why are we still using ECT?," 2013).

As I stated earlier, this approach for the remediation of refractory depression is used to manage cases that do not respond to adequate courses of at least two antidepressants. ECT continues to have its supporters and detractors who concur that they do not understand the mechanism that creates the change effect in ECT.

Typically, insurance plans will pay for this intervention, which will typically incur the cost of a one-week hospital stay plus approximately $2,500 per session for at least ten sessions. Relapse is possible without maintenance treatments.

Another treatment available for medication resistant depression is called Transcranial Magnetic Stimulation (TMS) which is a noninvasive method used to cause depolarization or hyperpolarization in the neurons of the brain. TMS uses electromagnetic induction to induce weak electric currents using a rapidly changing magnetic field. The generation of a magnetic field by an electric current happens in accord with Ampere's Law, which says that the integral of the magnetizing field around any closed loop of the field is equal to the sum of the current flowing through the loop. This is how electric motors work. Conversely, an oscillating magnetic field can generate an electric current in a conductor such as a copper wire or the saltwater environment in the brain.

According to the United States National Institute of Mental Health, "TMS uses a magnet instead of an electrical current to activate the brain. An electromagnetic coil is held against the forehead and short electromagnetic pulses are administered through the coil. The magnetic pulse passes easily through the skull, and causes small electrical currents that stimulate nerve cells in the targeted brain region."

Because this type of pulse generally does not reach further than two inches into the brain, scientists can select which parts of the brain will be affected and which will not be. The magnetic field is about the same strength as that of a magnetic resonance imaging (MRI) scan. A variant of TMS, repetitive Transcranial Magnetic Stimulation (rTMS), has been tested as a treatment tool for various neurological and   psychiatric disorders. ("Brain Stimulation Therapies,")

A *New York Times* article on the use of transcranial magnetic stimulation was featured with regard to a "treatment-resistant depression" patient. As reported:

"Martha Rhodes experienced her first bout of depression at 13. By her late 50s, she had taken just about every antidepressant there is, including Zoloft, Lexapro and Paxil— which did the trick for many years, but had side effects — then Effexor, Lamictal, Seroquel and Abilify.

"After a suicide attempt in 2009, she tried something radically different: transcranial magnetic stimulation. . . Every day, she spent just over half an hour in a chair with a powerful magnet affixed to the front left side of her head. After four weeks, "I woke up and something was different," said Mrs. Rhodes, who wrote a book, *3,000 Pulses Later*, describing the treatment. "I felt lighter. I didn't wake up in the morning and wish I were dead."

. . . While it's fairly clear that TMS is effective in some percentage of patients with major depressive disorder, it's still not very easy to know in advance who those patients are," said Dr. Steven J. Zalcman, the head of the clinical neuroscience research branch of the National Institute of Mental Health. The American Psychiatric Association's practice guidelines say that TMS confers "relatively small to moderate benefits," and the results of clinical trials have been decidedly mixed.

The glass is half full or half empty, depending on where you're coming from," said Dr. Mark S. George, a professor at the Medical University of South Carolina in Charleston. A randomized trial of repetitive TMS to treat resistant depression was used with the study results finding that nearly three times as many patients went into remission after TMS treatment, compared with those receiving a placebo.

"The absolute numbers were still small: Only 14 percent of treated patients recovered, compared with 5 percent in the placebo group. A newer variation of the treatment, deep TMS, was developed by an Israeli company called Brainsway and approved by the Food and Drug Administration this year (2014)." (Rabin, 1372713639)

Cost aspects of TMS vary with a range of $400 to $500 per session being typical. A total cost is around

$15,000, with some insurance companies beginning to cover the expenses. Scalp irritation or headaches are the most common side effects.

Typically, a 50-minute session is required, best provided on a daily basis including weekends for 3 to 5 weeks. It seems as though the risk for this non-medication-responsive patient group includes risky, quite expensive and time consuming intervention with little scientific backup or rationale.

Another emerging treatment actually involves an implant placed in the chest area, which is designed to send an electrical impulse to the vagus nerve for 30 seconds every 5 minutes. It is typically kept inside the body for 10 weeks or more and then removed. Its first use was to help stabilize epilepsy, but it was applied next to patients with treatment-resistant depression. At present, it is limited to persons who are 18 years of age or older with the surgery usually requiring a 30 to 60-minute intervention. (Critchley et al., 2007)

Limited research has found no effect on targeted chronic depression. Negative side effects include vocal changes, coughing, potential numbness of skin in the treated region, and shortness of breath. It may take 6 to 12 months to become aware of any benefits of this specific intervention. It is likely not covered by most insurance plans including Medicare. The cost factor ranges from $10,000 to $20,000.

A 2007 article suggests a shift in thinking related to our perception of the specific circuitry in the brain that mediates depression. The authors reported that:

". . . Several lines of evidence suggest that there are specific neural circuits within the limbic-cortical system that mediate stress-responsiveness, mood and emotional regulation. Disorders of mood and anxiety represent brain-based disorders that lead to dysregulation of these circuits. Traditional psychiatric medication, psychotherapy and somatic therapies converge in bringing homeostasis to these disrupted circuits.

"New neuro-stimulatory therapies based on progress in understanding emotion circuitry and new pharmacological therapies based on understanding emotional learning are likely to provide more rapid and robust methodologies for treating these debilitating and complex disorders." (Ressler & Mayberg, 2007)

Summary

There is now little question that PTSD and varied forms of depression co-occur with much frequency. If a number assists in illustrating the relationship, one is safe with the 50% figure, wherein for every two

Veterans diagnosed with PTSD, one is likely to have a comorbid diagnosis of depression.

The diagnosis of treatment-resistant depression is invoked when a patient is non-responsive to one or two courses of anti-depressant medication. I find it incomprehensible that it is estimated that 271,000 Vietnam theater veterans continue to suffer from full blown PTSD symptoms with one-third continuing to have current major depressive disorder. I view this group as being an at-risk population that has remained silent and endured their internalized and hidden wounds of war for decades.

Among the newer generation of Veterans, those who served and have both disorders (PTSD and MDD) were almost three times more likely to report suicidality within the past year than those with either diagnosis alone. Veterans who have used an urgent care psychiatric clinic and completed a survey specified that "More than half the sample (52%) reported suicidal ideation during the prior week. Of these, more than one-third (37%) had active ideation which included participants with a current suicide plan (27%) and those who had made preparations to carry out their plan (12%)."

I reviewed briefly the economic costs of depression. A brain structure called the Lateral Habenula (LHb) was introduced and described as being associated with both excitatory and inhibitory neurons. I noted that too much excitement in this structure is associated with depression, while diminished activity is linked with sensations ranging from contentment to joy. Targeting this structure provides an opportunity to remediate depression in a manner similar to ECT, free of ECT's potential deleterious side-effects.

I described the use of RESET-Depression, also referred to as the Disappointment/Despair/Depression circuit (3-D's), along with the steps used with BAUD to target this brain structure. A case study was provided to exemplify the procedure. I also reviewed and discussed alternative current interventions for treatment resistant depression.

I provided a final comment pertaining to a shift in thinking about depression as being a circuit disorder occurring within the limbic-cortical system as opposed to being a condition of unknown origin.

Reference List:

Aiyer, R., & Joffe, R. T. (2015). Deep Brain Stimulation in Treatment Resistant Depression: A Systematic Review. *Current Psychopharmacology, 4*(1), 10–16.

Andrade, C. (2014). A primer for the conceptualization of the mechanism of action of electroconvulsive therapy, 1: defining the question. *The Journal of Clinical Psychiatry,*

75(5), e410-412. https://doi.org
/10.4088/JCP.14f09185

Brain Stimulation Therapies. https://www.nimh.
nih.gov/health/topics/brain-stimulation-
therapies/brain-stimulation-therapies.shtml

Canu, E., Kostić, M., Agosta, F., Munjiza, A.,
Ferraro, P. M., Pesic, D., ... Filippi, M.
(2015). Brain structural abnormalities in
patients with major depression with or
without generalized anxiety disorder
comorbidity. *Journal of Neurology, 262*(5),
1255–1265. https://doi.org/10.1007/s00415-
015-7701-z

Cleary, D. R., Ozpinar, A., Raslan, A. M., & Ko, A.
L. (2015). Deep brain stimulation for
psychiatric disorders: where we are now.
Neurosurgical Focus, 38(6), E2.
https://doi.org/10.3171/2015.3.FOCUS1546

Critchley, H. D., Lewis, P. A., Orth, M., Josephs, O.,
Deichmann, R., Trimble, M. R., & Dolan, R.
J. (2007). Vagus nerve stimulation for treat
ment-resistant depression: behavioral and
neural effects on encoding negative material.
Psychosomatic Medicine, 69(1), 17–22.
https://doi.org/10.1097/PSY.0b013e31802e10
6d

Flory, J. D., & Yehuda, R. (2015). Comorbidity
between post-traumatic stress disorder and
major depressive disorder: alternative
explanations and treatment considerations.

Dialogues in Clinical Neuroscience, 17(2), 141–150.

Fosse, R., & Read, J. (2013). Electroconvulsive Treatment: Hypotheses about Mechanisms of Action. *Frontiers in Psychiatry, 4*. https://doi.org/10.3389/fpsyt.2013.00094

Greenberg, P. E., Fournier, A.-A., Sisitsky, T., Pike, C. T., & Kessler, R. C. (2015). The Economic Burden of Adults With Major Depressive Disorder in the United States (2005 and 2010). *The Journal of Clinical Psychiatry,* 155–162. https://doi.org/10.4088/JCP.14m09298

Hsu, Y.-W. A., Wang, S. D., Wang, S., Morton, G., Zariwala, H. A., Iglesia, H. O. de la, & Turner, E. E. (2014). Role of the Dorsal Medial Habenula in the Regulation of Voluntary Activity, Motor Function, Hedonic State, and Primary Reinforcement. *The Journal of Neuroscience, 34*(34), 11366–11384. https://doi.org/10.1523/JNEUROSCI.1861-14.2014

Juckel, G., Uhl, I., Padberg, F., Brüne, M., & Winter, C. (2009). Psychosurgery and deep brain stimulation as ultima ratio treatment for refractory depression. *European Archives of Psychiatry and Clinical Neuroscience, 259*(1), 1–7. https://doi.org/10.1007/s00406-008-0826-7

Kessler, R. C., Berglund, P., Demler, O., Jin, R.,
Koretz, D., Merikangas, K. R., … National
Comorbidity Survey Replication. (2003). The
epidemiology of major depressive disorder:
results from the National Comorbidity Survey
Replication (NCS-R). *JAMA, 289*(23), 3095–
3105. https://doi.org/10.1001
/jama.289.23.3095

Lenze, E., Blumberger, D. M., Karp, J. F., &
Reynolds, C. F. (2015). Treatment-Resistant
Depression in Late-Life: New Research
Findings. *The American Journal of Geriatric
Psychiatry, 23*(3), S10–S11. https://doi.org
/10.1016/j.jagp.2014.12.017

Levine, P. A. (2010). *In an Unspoken Voice: How the
Body Releases Trauma and Restores
Goodness*. North Atlantic Books.

Maguen, S., Metzler, T. J., Bosch, J., Marmar, C. R.,
Knight, S. J., & Neylan, T. C. (2012). Killing
in combat may be independently associated
with suicidal ideation. *Depression and
Anxiety, 29*(11), 918–923. https://doi.org
/10.1002/da.21954

Marmar, C. R., Schlenger, W., Henn-Haase, C., Qian,
M., Purchia, E., Li, M., … Kulka, R. A.
(2015). Course of Posttraumatic Stress
Disorder 40 Years After the Vietnam War:
Findings From the National Vietnam Veterans
Longitudinal Study. *JAMA Psychiatry, 72*(9),

875–881. https://doi.org/10.1001/jama
psychiatry.2015.0803

McClure, J. R., Criqui, M. H., Macera, C. A., Ji, M.,
Nievergelt, C. M., & Zisook, S. (2015).
Prevalence of suicidal ideation and other
suicide warning signs in veterans attending an
urgent care psychiatric clinic. *Comprehensive
Psychiatry*, *60*, 149–155. https://doi.org
/10.1016/j.comppsych.2014.09.010

Proulx, C. D., Hikosaka, O., & Malinow, R. (2014).
Reward processing by the lateral habenula in
normal and depressive behaviors. *Nature
Neuroscience*, *17*(9), 1146–1152.
https://doi.org/10.1038/nn.3779

PTSD: Brain On Fire. https://www.academia.edu
/19524765/PTSD_Brain_On_Fire

Purse, M. Experiences With ECT - Electroconvulsive
Therapy. https://www.verywell.com
/experiences-with-ect-electroconvulsive-
therapy-379902

Rabin, R. C. (1372713639). New Approach to
Depression. *Well*. http://well.blogs.nytimes
.com/2013/07/01/new-approach-to-
depression/

Ramsawh, H. J., Fullerton, C. S., Mash, H. B. H., Ng,
T. H. H., Kessler, R. C., Stein, M. B., &
Ursano, R. J. (2014). Risk for suicidal
behaviors associated with PTSD, depression,
and their comorbidity in the U.S. Army.

Journal of Affective Disorders, *161*, 116–122.
https://doi.org/10.1016/j.jad.2014.03.016

Ressler, K. J., & Mayberg, H. S. (2007). Targeting
abnormal neural circuits in mood and anxiety
disorders: from the laboratory to the clinic.
Nature Neuroscience, *10*(9), 1116–1124.
https://doi.org/10.1038/nn1944

Ryder, J. G., & Holtzheimer, P. E. (2016). Deep
Brain Stimulation for Depression: An Update.
Current Behavioral Neuroscience Reports,
3(2), 102–108. https://doi.org/
10.1007/s40473-016-0073-6

Rytwinski, N. K., Scur, M. D., Feeny, N. C., &
Youngstrom, E. A. (2013). The co-occurrence
of major depressive disorder among
individuals with posttraumatic stress disorder:
a meta-analysis. *Journal of Traumatic Stress*,
26(3), 299–309. https://doi.org
/10.1002/jts.21814

Sartorius, A., Kiening, K. L., Kirsch, P., Gall, C. C.
von, Haberkorn, U., Unterberg, A. W., …
Meyer-Lindenberg, A. (2010). Remission of
Major Depression Under Deep Brain
Stimulation of the Lateral Habenula in a
Therapy-Refractory Patient. *Biological
Psychiatry*, *67*(2), e9–e11. https://doi.org
/10.1016/j.biopsych.2009.08.027

Thase, M. E. (2011). Treatment-resistant depression:
prevalence, risk factors, and treatment
strategies. *The Journal of Clinical Psychiatry*,

72(5), e18. https://doi.org/10.4088
/JCP.8133tx4c

Treatment for Depression After Unsatisfactory
Response to SSRIs - Executive Summary |
AHRQ Effective Health Care Program. http://
effectivehealthcare.ahrq.gov/index.cfm/search
-for-guides-reviews-and-reports/?page
action=displayproduct&productid=1036

Tylee, A., Gastpar, M., Lépine, J. P., & Mendlewicz,
J. (1999). Identification of depressed patient
types in the community and their treatment
needs: findings from the DEPRES II
(Depression Research in European Society II)
survey. DEPRES Steering Committee.
International Clinical Psychopharmacology,
14(3), 153–165.

Why are we still using ECT? (2013, July 24). *BBC
News*. http://www.bbc.co.uk/news/health-
23414888

Chapter Five:

SURVIVOR'S GUILT
& MORAL INJURY

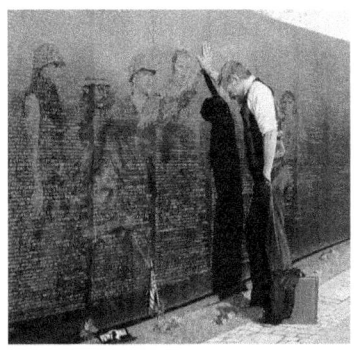

"At some of the darkest moments in my life, some people I thought of as friends deserted me-some because they cared about me and it hurt them to see me in pain; others because I reminded them of their own vulnerability, and that was more than they could handle. But real friends overcame their discomfort and came to sit with me. If they had not words to make me feel better, they sat in silence (much better than saying, "You'll get over it," or "It's not so bad; others have it worse") and I loved them for it."

Harold Kushner, Living a Life that Matters

As noted in the following article, reference is made to "Survivor Guilt" where it is stated:

> Individuals may experience survivor guilt following casualties during which fellow service members are severely wounded or killed, or when they are at home while their unit is deployed. Individuals coping with survivor guilt may find themselves wondering questions such as:
>
> 1) "Why didn't I get hurt?"
> 2) "Why did I live when other people died?"
> 3) "What could I have done differently to prevent it?" ("Traumatic Brain Injury,")

I will interweave historical (with thanks to Dr. Jonathan Shay) and current examples of survivor's guilt and moral injury throughout the ensuing discussion separating the inserts by asterisks.

In *The Iliad*, Homer's main character, Achilles, became beleaguered with feelings of grief upon being informed of the death of Patroclus. He experienced 'survivor's guilt' with intrusive thoughts that disturbed his sleep:

****

> ...but Achilles still wept for thinking of his dear comrade, and sleep, before whom all

things bow, could take no hold upon him. . .
As he dwelt on these things he wept bitterly
and lay now on his side, now on his back, and
now face downwards, till at last he rose and
went out as one distraught to wander upon the
sea-shore.

I would die here and now, in that I could not
save my comrade. He has fallen far from
home, and in his hour of need my hand was
not there to help him. What is there for me?
Return to my own land I shall not, and I have
brought no saving neither to Patroclus nor to
my other comrades of whom so many have
been slain by mighty Hector; I stay here by
my ships a bootless burden upon the earth.
(Kucmin, Kucmin, Nogalski, Sojczuk, &
Jojczuk, 2016).

****

As a relatively new author, I found that searching for
recent and pertinent material can at times be a
daunting task. Through my first cursory review of the
material, I chose 12 articles to begin with and then, I
struck the motherlode. As this goldmine of material is
provided through the U. S. Department of Veteran
Affairs (VA), it is unrestricted with regard to the
relevant data that can be copied and discussed.

In addition to the VA data, I've utilized material from psychologist Dr. Ilona Pivar whose material is contained within the article. Although I've moved some of Dr. Pivar's material around in this discussion, the information she's provided is basically unedited. ("Iraq War Clinician Guide - 2nd Edition - PTSD,") My plan is to use Dr. Pivar's perspective as a comprehensive foundation about the topic of survivor's guilt.

I begin with differentiating grief from depression and PTSD. This is followed by Dr. Pivar's definitions of different aspects of guilt/grief. Next, Dr. Pivar breaks out material specifically related to Vietnam Veterans and Iraq Veterans. Finally, I've included her thoughts in regards to assessing and treating traumatic guilt in returning Veterans. We will begin with the differentiation issue with Dr. Pivar stating that:

"Although research into the prevalence and intensity of grief symptoms in war veterans is limited, clinicians recognize the importance for veterans of grieving the loss of comrades. Grief symptoms can include sadness, longing, missing the deceased, non-acceptance of the death, feeling the death was unfair, anger, feeling stunned, dazed, or shocked, emptiness, preoccupation with thoughts and images of the deceased, loss of enjoyment, difficulties in trusting others, social impairments, and guilt concerning the circumstances of the death.

"Recent research results, although limited to one sample of Vietnam combat veterans in a residential rehabilitation unit for PTSD, have supported findings in the general bereavement literature that unresolved grief can be detected as a distress syndrome distinct from depression and anxiety. In this sample of combat veterans, grief symptoms were detected at very high levels of intensity, thirty years' post-loss.

"The intensity of symptoms experienced after thirty years was similar to that reported in community samples of grieving spouses and parents at six months' post-loss. This supports clinical observations that unresolved grief, if left untreated, can continue unabated and increases the distress load of veterans. The existence of a distinct and intense set of grief symptoms indicates the need for clinical attention to grief in the treatment plan." ("Iraq War Clinician Guide - XI. Traumatic Grief: - iraq_clinician_guide _ch_11 .pdf,")

Dr. Pivar next discusses the issue of normal grieving versus the emergence of a pathological grief process Apparently, the differentiation between the normal versus pathological states is a time continent variable apparently based upon a six-month variable that is not associated with the symptom picture itself, other than the fact that the intensity does not dissipate over time. She notes:

"Bereavement is a universal experience. Intense emotions, including sadness, longing, anger, and guilt, are reactions to the loss of a close person. Common in the first days and weeks of grieving are intense emotions, usually experienced as coming in waves lasting 20 minutes to an hour, with accompanying somatic sensations in the stomach, tightness in the throat, shortness of breath, intense fatigue, feeling faint, agitation, and helplessness.

"Lack of motivation, loss of interest in outside activities, and social withdrawal are also fairly common. A person experiencing normal grief will have a gradual decline in symptoms and distress. When grief symptoms remain at severely discomforting levels, even after two months, a referral to a clinician can be considered.

"If intense symptoms persist after six months, a diagnosis of complicated grief can be made and there is a definite indication for clinical intervention. Complicated grief prolonged over time has been shown to have negative effects on health, social functioning, and mental health." ("Iraq War

Clinician Guide - XI. Traumatic Grief: - iraq_clinician _guide_ch_11.pdf ,")

The unknown author of an epic from the third millennium B.C. of the legendary king of the city of Ung, describes Gilgamesh's despair and the consequences of witnessing the violent death of his companion Enkidu, who was killed in a battle. Gilgamesh suffers from recurring intrusive memories regarding Enkidu's death and asks numerous questions regarding his own death:

****

I wept for him seven days and nights till the worm fastened on him. Because of my brother I am afraid of death, because of my brother I stray through the wilderness. His fate lies heavy upon me. How can I be silent, how can I rest? He is dust and I too shall die and be laid in the earth for ever. I am afraid of death (Kucmin et al., 2016)."

****

An acute reaction can occur which can overlay normative grief with this consequence referred to as Acute Traumatic Grief. Dr. Pivar suggests that adding trauma to the mix can exacerbate the underlying grief process thereby magnifying the symptomology:

"Survivors of traumatic events can experience acute symptoms of distress including intense agitation, self-accusations, high-risk behaviors, suicidal ideation, and intense outbursts of anger, superimposed on the symptoms of normal bereavement.

"Soldiers who lose their comrades in battle have been known to make heroic efforts to save them or recover their bodies. Some soldiers have reacted with rage at the enemy, risking their lives with little thought ("gone berserk" or "kill crazy").

"Some soldiers withdraw and become loners, seldom or never again making friends; some express extreme anger at the events and personnel that brought them to the conflict. Some soldiers are inclined to mask their emotions. Any sign of vulnerability or "losing" it can indicate that they are not tough enough to handle combat.

"Delaying grief may well postpone problems that can become chronic symptoms weeks, months and years later. The returning veteran who has developed PTSD and/or depression may well be masking his or her grief symptoms." ("Iraq War Clinician Guide - XI. Trauma-tic Grief: - iraq_clinician _guide_ch_11.pdf ,")

Dr. Pivar discussed traumatic grief in a context different from the acute reaction type. My understanding is that she is discussing the causative aspect rather than the suddenness-of-onset factor. She defines traumatic grief as:

"The experience of the sudden loss of a significant and close attachment. Having a close buddy, identification with soldiers in the unit, and experiencing multiple losses were the strongest predictors of grief symptoms.

"Factors important . . . may include exposure to significant numbers of civilian casualties, exposure to death from friendly fire or accidents resulting from massive and rapid troop movements, and concern about culpability for having caused death or harm to civilians in cities. These factors may contribute to experiences of shock, disbelief, and self-blame that increase risk of traumatic and complicated grief reactions." ("Iraq War Clinician Guide - XI. Traumatic Grief: - iraq_clinician_guide_ch_11.pdf,")

****

I'm guilty all my life. I'm guilty I didn't save my father, my mother, my sister. I feel guilty, I could have made Aryan papers for them. I'm guilty I tried to talk them into going to Russia, but they wouldn't listen. I'm guilty, I don't want to be richer than my father. I had opportunities to make millions. I always feel guilty. Why should I have more than my parents? Maybe I'm wrong. I'm guilty. I feel guilty all my life.

In December 1944, when the war started coming to an end, although we didn't know that, or we did not know to what extent — we were taken out of camp and started off to march — the Russians came near and the Germans took us out from camp and they marched us to other camps.

It was terrible cold; we had no clothes. Whoever could not walk they shot. We had no food. At night they herded us in some farm… a barn. Next morning very early they took us out and we had to march again; we marched for days. And during the march, my brother… he could not walk anymore and he was taken from me and shot on the road.

It is difficult to say, [to] talk about feelings. First of all, we were reduced to such an animal level that actually now that I remember those things, I feel more horrible than I felt at the time. We were in such a state that all that mattered is to remain alive. Even about your own brother, one did not think. I don't know how other people felt...

It bothers me very much if I was the only one that felt that way, or is that normal in such circumstances to be that way? I feel now sometimes, did I do my best or didn't I do something that I should have done? But at the time I wanted to survive myself, and maybe I did not give my greatest efforts to do certain things, or I missed to do certain things (Langer, 1991)."

****

The topic of assessing and treating acute grief in returning Veterans needs to be addressed in its own right. Unfortunately, the reality is that when large numbers of individuals who have likely been involved in multiple tours of service are rotated back, identifying individual symptomology is likely to be an impossible task. Dr. Pivar noted that:

"Clinical judgment is necessary in deciding when and how to treat acute grief reactions, especially when they are accompanied by a diagnosis of acute stress disorder. While a cognitive-behavioral treatment package that includes exposure therapy has been shown to prevent the development of PTSD in some persons with acute stress disorder, exposure therapy during the initial stages of grief may often be contraindicated, because it may place great emotional strain on someone only just bereaved.

"Bereavement researchers also are hesitant to treat grief in the first few months of a normal loss, wishing not to interfere with a natural healing process. In the early stages of grief, symptoms may be experienced as intense, but this is normal for the first days, weeks, and months. Soldiers surviving a traumatic loss in the war zone will be more likely to mask intense feelings of sadness, pain, vulnerability, anxiety, anger, and guilt.

"Balancing other traumatic experiences with the intensity of grief may feel overwhelming. Therefore, it is important to assess and respect the individual soldier's ability to cope and manage these feelings at any time.

"A soldier may be relieved to know that someone understands how he or she feels after losing a buddy, or experiencing other losses including civilians or multiple deaths in the field, and communication with a clinician may be a first step in coming to terms with loss. However, that soldier may not be ready to probe more deeply into feelings and circumstances. Care and patience in the assessment process, as well as in beginning treatment, is essential.

"Treatment during the acute stages of grief would best include acknowledgement of the loss, communication of understanding of the depth of feelings, encour-agement to recover positive memories of the deceased, recognition of the good intentions of the survivor to come to the aid of the deceased, education about what to expect during the course of acute grief, and encouragement of distraction and relaxation techniques as a temporary palliative.

"Efforts to reduce symptoms of PTSD and depression as co-morbid disorders would take precedence over grief symptoms in the initial phases of treatment, unless the loss itself is the main cause of distress." ("Iraq War Clinician Guide - XI. Traumatic Grief: - iraq_clinician_guide_ch_11.pdf,")

My curious nature leads me to question, is there truly a difference between PTSD and Survivor's Guilt/Traumatic Grief Reaction? Following the rules of parsimony, if the long-term symptoms are identical and respond in a similar method to treatment intervention, I would speculate that the same neural circuitry is involved. In other words, if it quacks, waddles and looks like a duck, it's a duck!

My clinical experience as exemplified in my first book, *Ending the Nightmare of PTSD*, Chapter One, illustrated this point in my case study of a Veteran with survivor's guilt. Shawn O'Hara's survivor's guilt symptoms went into full remission with one RESET Therapy treatment session.

Thus, unless proven otherwise, I believe that the two conditions share the same neural circuitry. If this proves to be the case, prolonging treatment for an extended period of time (up to six months) is a disservice to the Veteran with the condition. We now shift to review Dr. Pivar's specific reference to Vietnam Veterans. She noted that:

". . . The sudden loss of attachments takes many forms in the war zone. Soldiers may experience overwhelming self-blame for events that are not under their control, including deaths during the chaos of firefights, accidents and failures of equipment, medical triage, and casualties from friendly fire.

"The everyday infantryman from Vietnam lived his mistakes over and over again, perhaps in order to find some way of relieving pain and guilt from the death of friends. Many medics during Vietnam suffered tremendously when they were not able to save members of their unit, especially when they identified strongly with the men under their care. Pilots called in to fire close to troops were overcome with guilt when their ordinance hit American soldiers even while saving a majority of men.

"Officers felt unique responsibility for the subordinates under their care and suffered undue guilt and grief when results of combat were damaging. Soldiers who worked closely with civilians were often shocked when they witnessed deaths of people with whom they had come to develop mutual trust. Deaths of civilian women and children were difficult to bear.

"Bonds with unit members are described by many veterans as some of the closest relationships they have formed in their lives. During Vietnam, soldiers were rotated in and out of units on individual schedules. Nevertheless, the percentage of returning veterans with PTSD who also report bereavement-related distress is high." ("Iraq War Clinician Guide - XI. Traumatic Grief: - iraq_clinician _guide_ch_11.pdf ,")

We will now strategically shift to Dr. Pivar's material specifically pertaining to the Iraq conflict:

"In the Iraq conflict, young soldiers and reservists have remained with their units throughout training and deployment. Levels of mutual trust and respect, unit cohesiveness, and affective bonding will have been further strengthened by the experiences of deployment.

"While bonding and attachment to the unit may result in some protection against subsequent development of PTSD, unresolved bereavement may be expected to be associated with increased distress over the life span unless these losses are acknowledged and grief symptoms treated on a timely basis." ("Iraq War Clinician Guide - XI. Traumatic Grief: - iraq_clinician_guide_ch_11.pdf,")

Dr. Pivar's discussion of grief ends with material pertaining to her perception of intervention strategies for returning Veterans. She advises that:

". . . Clinical experience supports the importance of education about normal and complicated grief processes, education about the cognitive processes of guilt, restructuring of cognitive distortions of events that might lead to excessive guilt, looking at the function of anger in bereavement, restoring positive memories of the deceased, restoration and acknowledgment of caring feelings towards the deceased, affirming resilience and positive coping, retelling the story of the death, and learning to tolerate painful feelings as part of the grieving process.

"These activities can be provided in individual treatment or in closed groups. Regardless of the techniques that are used, what is central to treating veterans for prolonged and complicated grief is recognition of the significance of their losses, provision of an opportunity to talk about the deceased, restructuring of distorted thoughts of guilt, and validation of the pain and intensity of their feelings. What is most essential is that bereavement and loss be treated in addition to PTSD and depression for a more complete recovery.

"Grief symptoms including sadness, distress, guilt, anger, intrusive thoughts, and preoccupation with the death should be declining after about six months during a normal grieving process. If symptoms remain very high after six months; clinical intervention is warranted." ("Iraq War Clinician Guide - XI. Traumatic Grief: - iraq_clinician _guide_ch_11.pdf,")

While I am in agreement that bereavement issues should be treated in a manner similar to that of PTSD and depression, I simultaneously hold the belief that none of our current, mainstream treatment options effectively remediate the described conditions.

I've clearly taken the position that education has no positive effect whatsoever on trauma-altered limbic circuitry. Nor does 'retelling the story' repeatedly, as called for in Prolonged Exposure Therapy, signifi-cantly alter the trauma network.

In my mind, group therapy processes come after the neuronal circuit has been RESET, not before. Until Executive Functioning is reestablished in the pre-frontal lobes, vocalization of traumatic experiences from others in the group simply reaffirms to the collective limbic brains that the world is a dangerous and treacherous place.

Thus, it is my position that, 'what is essential' is the restoration of pre-trauma, pre-grief functioning in the afflicted Veteran to facilitate the opportunity to revert from a protective, defensive mode to a growth opportunity. Only after a successful reset experience has occurred can the Veteran truly benefit from the potential of meaningful interaction with his or her comrades within the group therapy setting. We will now shift to the topic of Moral Injury (MI), which is described as being:

"characterized by guilt, existential crisis, and loss of trust that may develop following a perceived moral violation. The present article reviews phenomen-ological descriptions, incidence, etiology, and symptoms of moral injury, with a view toward providing an updated conceptual definition.

"Moral injury's existing definition (Litz et al., 2009) is updated to emphasize its empirically and theoretically recognized symptoms. Guilt, shame, spiritual/ existential conflict, and loss of trust are identified as core symptoms. Depression, anxiety, anger, re-experiencing, self-harm, and social problems are identified as secondary symptoms." (Jinkerson, 2016)

****

The dead soldier takes his misery with him, but the man who killed him must forever live and die with him. The lesson becomes increasingly clear: Killing is what war is all about, and killing in combat, by its very nature, causes deep wounds of pain and guilt. The language of war helps us deny what war is really about, and in doing so makes war more palatable." ("Microsoft Word - Moral Injury (1).docx - jpj_moral_injury.pdf,")

****

America claims innocence and goodness as fundamental traits. We believe that our young men and women should be able to go to war, get the job done, and return home blameless as well. That is how quintessential American hero, John Wayne, portrayed the experience of warfare to generations. Many Vietnam War veterans referred to him as a guiding image (Tick, 2012)."

The author of a 2010 article recognized the impact of killing in combat, during the Iraq War, as

". . . a significant indicator of mental health problems with an association between killing and the desire to engage in self-harm. A previous study found similar outcomes, including symptoms of PTSD, dissociation, functional impairment, and violent behaviors. This study concluded that veteran experiences of killing in war are crucial considerations for the evaluation and treatment of veterans." ("Moral Injury in Veterans of War - v23n1.pdf,")

Additional comment on this material follows:

"While guilt has been recognized as part of PTSD, shame is usually ignored. These feelings are related to not only suicide, but to relationship problems, domestic violence and dramatic increase in use of substances such as alcohol. They are also related to the phenomena of veterans entering the criminal justice system following discharge from the military.

"It must be pointed out that the vast majority of veterans had no criminal history prior to entering the military and that most veterans do not experience judicial or non-judicial punishment during the period they serve in the military." ("Microsoft Word - Moral Injury (1).docx - jpj_moral_injury.pdf,")

Many combat veterans, particularly those who served in infantry units during war, would agree that the experiences they incurred were often attributed to luck. If no one in your unit was injured or killed during an operation it was considered good luck.

If someone was injured or killed it was often attributed to bad luck. On page 30 in his excellent 1994 book, *Achilles in Vietnam*, Dr. Jonathan Shay covered this issue, and coined the term "Moral Luck." Shay uses the statements of two Vietnam veterans in group therapy to portray what he means by moral luck. The first veteran who experienced bad luck stated:

"Well, at first, I mean when I first come there, I couldn't believe what I was seeing. I couldn't believe Americans could do things like that to another human being ... but then I became that. We went through villages and killed everything. I mean everything, and that was all right with me." (Litz et al., 2009)

****

Shifting now to the issue of 'Moral Injury,' the modern use of the term was attributed to Dr. Shay (Shay and Munroe, 1998). The authors wrote that the current definition of moral injury has three parts:

Moral injury is present when (1) there has been a betrayal of what is morally correct; (2) by someone who holds legitimate authority; and (3) in a high-stakes situation.

Further development of this concept has been credited to Brett Litz and colleagues who define moral injury as:

". . . perpetrating, failing to prevent, bearing witness to, or learning about acts that transgress deeply held moral beliefs and expectations." (Litz et al., 2009)

They propose a conceptual model based on cognitive dissonance which occurs:

"after a perceived moral transgression resulting in stable internal global attributions of blame, followed by the experience of shame, guilt, or anxiety, causing the individual to withdraw from others. The result is increased risk of suicide due to demoralization, self-harming, and self-handicapping behaviors.

"Throughout history, warriors have been confronted with moral and ethical challenges and modern unconventional and guerilla wars amplify these challenges. Potentially morally injurious events, such as perpetrating, failing to prevent, or bearing witness to acts that transgress deeply held moral beliefs and expectations may be deleterious in the long-term, emotionally, psychologically, behaviorally, spiritually, and socially (what we label as moral injury). Although there has been some research on the consequences of unnecessary acts of violence in war zones, the lasting impact of morally injurious experience in war remains chiefly unaddressed." (Litz et al., 2009)

William B. Brown speculates that:

"Defeating and killing the enemy is one of the fundamental goals or purposes of the military training curriculum. As noted by Brock and Lettini: Combatants who support a war and serve willingly also experience moral injury because the actual conditions of war are morally anguishing.

"As every veteran of combat knows, the ideal of war service, the glamor of its heroics, and the training for killing fail to prepare warriors for the true horrors and moral atrocities (2012, p. xvii). When asked to describe the primary thing they learned in Basic Training or Boot Camp, the most prevalent response was "weapons proficiency" followed by "defeat or kill the enemy." ("Microsoft Word - Moral Injury (1).docx - jpj_moral_injury.pdf,")

The topic of luck in war expands beyond the Vietnam War to the more recent wars in Afghanistan and Iraq. It also stretches far beyond the witnessing or not witnessing of horrific events in war.

Sherman (2015) discusses the experiences of a Noncommissioned Officer (NCO) who served in Iraq, points out that the NCO was ordered to take a couple days of Rest and Relaxation (R and R) in Qatar.

"The NCO's primary duties included providing intelligence regarding geographic and cultural information pertaining to his unit's Area of Operation AO)." ("Microsoft Word - Moral Injury (1).docx - jpj_moral_injury.pdf,")

****

Shortly after arriving in Qatar he heard that members of his unit were in a vehicle that had hit an IED (Improvised Explosive Device) and that several soldiers had been killed in the explosion. The soldier felt that if he had been there the deaths might not have occurred. Hence, in the mind of this soldier, the deaths of his comrades were linked to luck. Had he not gone on R and R – had he remained in Iraq – the other soldiers might not have been killed.

Another Marine who was deployed to Iraq three times talks about the killing of an unarmed Iraqi woman by members of a marine unit:

I remember one woman walking by. She was carrying a huge bag, and she looked like she was heading toward us, so we lit her up with the Mark 19, which is an automatic grenade launcher, and when the dust settled, we realized the bag was filled with groceries. She had been trying to bring us food and we blew her to pieces." (Washburn, 2008), ("Microsoft Word - Moral Injury (1).docx - jpj_moral_ injury.pdf,")

****

Discussing one veteran's experiences in war, Shay notes that the veteran felt that he had become an evil person in Vietnam. As the veteran stated:

"Why I became like that? It was all evil. All evil. Where before, I wasn't. I look back. I look back today, and I am horrified at what I turned into. What I was. What I did. I just look at it like it was somebody else. I really do. It was somebody else.

"Somebody had control over me. War changes you, changes you. Strips you, strips you all of your beliefs, your religion, takes your dignity away, you become an animal." (1994, p. 33) ("Microsoft Word - Moral Injury (1).docx - jpj_moral_ injury.pdf,")

Shay further noted that this veteran had acquired a sense of revenge – it became the veteran's only value. All of his previous relationships no longer had meaning. He stopped writing home. The veteran told Shay that all he cared about was revenge. When the veteran returned home he said:

"I carried this home with me. I lost all of my friends, beat up my sister, went after my father. I mean, I just went after anybody and everything. Every three days I would totally explode; lose it for no reason at all. I'd be sitting there calm as could be, and this monster would come out of me with a fury that most people didn't want to be around. So it wasn't just over there [Vietnam]. I brought it back here with me." ("Microsoft Word - Moral Injury (1).docx - jpj_moral_ injury.pdf,")

There exists a clear distinction between individual morality and social morality. In the case of individual morality, we are referring to the basis from which individuals make judgments (e.g., loyalty, honesty, behaving responsibly, or acting in good faith). Individual morality includes perceptions of the principles of right and wrong relative to human behavior, and an individual's ethical and/or moral obligations to comply with that which he or she considers right.

"On the surface moral meaning or morality seems rather simple: always tell the truth, always treat others correctly, be respectable, always practice veracity, and always practice being virtuous to others, etc. We contend, however, that social morality is somewhat more complicated.

"Social morality outlines the basis of law that governs society and controls individual judgments and behavior. The principal focus of social morality is to insure the well-being of society. Society is larger than the individual, and individuals are part of society; people depend on society, but society also expects people to adhere to its rules and beliefs." (Collins, 1988) ("Microsoft Word - Moral Injury (1).docx - jpj_moral _injury.pdf,")

"Moral conflict can result when an individual's moral code is castigated by social moral paradoxes. For example, in American society seriously injuring or killing another human being is viewed as unconscionable or immoral in most instances, which is why we have laws that punish individuals for engaging in that behavior.

"On the other hand, American society readily accepts the killing and maiming of others in a conflict or war zone by American military personnel. Soldiers, sailors and air personnel worldwide find themselves in a difficult and contradictory position with regard to their moral identity.

"On the one hand, the instruments of violence bestow upon them awesome power. The implications of this responsibility have been dealt with extensively in the memoirs and auto-biographies of innumerable soldiers. Indeed, military personnel are subject, in conflict and war, to more wrenching emotional extremes than any other human profession. On the other hand, their relationship to the civilian authorities may be problematic - corruption, inefficiency and venality being prime causes for concern." (Williams, 1995, p. 5). ("Microsoft Word - Moral Injury (1).docx - jpj_moral_injury.pdf,")

"Moral Injury (MI) can be a violation of one's core cultural or spiritual values. MI can also be a violation of the soul. It has been suggested that MI is likely to be yet another signature wound of America's newest generation of veterans, and is very likely to result in lasting effects on veterans as well as their families." ("Microsoft Word - Moral Injury (1).docx - jpj_moral _injury.pdf,")

Finally, I will briefly explore a facet of MI that affects spiritual aspects of the afflicted individual.

The authors of the Coming Home Project suggest that:

> there is room to acknowledge the over-whelming psychic dilemmas that are best defined as spiritual injuries: guilt, anger and sadness that block peace of mind; the feeling that life no longer has meaning; and the bitter sense that God or life has let you down. ("Healing the Spiritual Wounds of War | Coming Home Project,")

Empirical evidence is inconsistent regarding the safeguard factor that religious belief offers in blocking against suicide ideation or attempts. The authors of the following article examined:

". . . positive and negative religious coping with risk for suicidal behavior in a sample of Iraq and/or Afghanistan Veterans. Participants completed self-report instruments assessing risk for suicidal behavior, religious coping, general combat exposure, morally injurious experiences, depression, and posttraumatic stress disorder (PTSD) symptoms. Frequency analyses revealed that half of all participants endorsed being religious, and adaptively drawing on religion to cope was more common than maladaptive coping.

"However, positive religious coping was not associated with suicidal behavior at the time of the study. In contrast, negative religious coping was uniquely associated with the risk for suicide when we controlled for demographic risk factors, war-zone experiences, depression, and PTSD.

"Although we expect adaptive reliance on religion to be beneficial for mental health, veterans who experience internal and/or external conflicts in the spiritual domain may be at increased risk for engaging in suicidal behavior following their war-zone service." (Currier, Smith, & Kuhlman, 2015).

Perhaps, we need to follow the way used for centuries by our native American tribes who had developed rituals and traditions for reintegrating their warriors upon returning to their communities.

"According to American Indian traditional beliefs, war affects a soldier's well-being, and makes it difficult for him to live in the everyday world. For American Indians, returning home means returning to a place—a land, a community, a family, and a culture—that you are part of, a place that you have a special relationship with.

"Participating in war interferes with your ability to be part of this place. It upsets the balance of life. This is why American Indian cultures have special ceremonies to help bring the soldier's life back into balance—to make it possible for the soldier to once again live in peace and to be physically, spiritually, emotionally, and mentally healthy.

"These ceremonies are part of the traditional religions of American Indians and are still part of life today for many American Indians. The ceremonies are powerful and have helped many Code Talkers and other returning soldiers. . .

"The Navajo people have different kinds of ceremonies for returning soldiers. When a soldier returns from war, his family can decide to sponsor a ceremony for him. They contact a spiritual leader, sometimes called a medicine man, who talks to the soldier about what he has experienced and decides which ceremony will be best for him. The Enemy Way ceremony, sometimes called the Squaw Dance, is one Navajo ceremony used for soldiers who were in combat, captured, or wounded.

"Intense preparations are made and, at the appropriate time, the ceremony is conducted. Often it includes family members and others who participate in the prayers, songs, and other parts of the ceremony. These ceremonies help the Navajo war veterans return to a state of balance, or beauty, within the universe. This state of balance is called "Hozho" in the Navajo language.

"I had nightmares thinking about the blood. The Japanese and the smell of the dead. Rotting Japanese and they probably got into my mind. And they had a Squaw Dance for me in Crystal. And I imagine they killed that evil spirit that was in my mind. That's what it's about. There's a lot of stories there. It takes a long time to talk about it. It usually takes a medicine man to explain everything properly. But it works.—John Brown, Jr., Navajo Code Talker, National Museum of the American Indian interview, 2004." ("Coming Home - Native Words Native Warriors,")."

Perhaps it is time for us to call for a national 'pow-wow' selecting the leaders among us from all corners of the nation to create our 'welcome home' rituals. It simply doesn't seem to be working to individually slip each of our current warriors into the mainstream of our society without recognizing the difficulties inherent in the transition.

Perhaps we need a personal guide akin to a 'medicine man' to facilitate the transformative journey. Given the multiple tours our Veterans experience in a dangerous world; they've earned the development of a better way to come home.

Summary

Clinically, I have challenged whether 'Survivor's Guilt' is a facet of the PTSD condition or, a distinct and separate disorder in its own right. My experience suggests that its traumatic presence alters brain circuitry in a similar fashion. Therapeutically, I have found it to reset to a growth mode rapidly through non-invasive, neuromodulation intervention.

I have issues with the suggested six-month wait period when it is proposed that the condition changes from that of a normal grieving process to that of a pathological grief process. I propose that delaying therapeutic intervention for this much time is not beneficial to the guilt-ridden Veteran.

Since I'm 'on a roll' here, I've also proposed that group therapy is not initially a treatment of choice for those who remain frozen in the protective/defensive mode. Rather, when the reset transformation occurs, bringing cognitive Executive Functioning back on line, this is the time that collegial support would be of benefit.

Within the context of material provided pertaining to 'Survivor's Guilt', comment was made regarding Veteran's in a residential rehabilitation unit still dealing with 30+ years of unresolved guilt. Personally, I'm inclined to take the position that anyone who has experienced combat or associated trauma would do best to 'detox' from the negative consequences of the experience. In order to do this, we would need an intervention that can rapidly and efficiently alter the likely negative outcome. To wait six-months to initiate effective change is an injustice to those who have served.

It would be best to accomplish this objective as early as possible such as when returning to base following an assignment. Notice that the term 'evaluation' is not being utilized here. The material provided in the chapter on dementia tells us that too many Veterans continue with the effects of PTSD over the course of a lifetime because their condition went undetected. Unfortunately, they have paid an enormous price in both their physical health and mental processing abilities.

A case example from my first book was provided to exemplify the means through which to accomplish the objective of resetting the neural circuitry that changes with the onset of trauma. Further comprehensive research is warranted to ascertain the efficacy of this approach.

Reference List:

Brown, W. B. Stanulis, R., & McElroy, G. (2016). Moral Injury as a collateral Damage Artifact of War in American Society: in Veterans of

War - Serving in war to serving time in jail and prison *Justice Policy Journal*, *13*(1), 1–41.

Coming Home - Native Words Native Warriors. http://nmai.si.edu/education/codetalkers/html/chapter5.html

Currier, J. M., Smith, P. N., & Kuhlman, S. (2015). Assessing the Unique Role of Religious Coping in Suicidal Behavior Among U.S. Iraq and Afghanistan Veterans. *Psychology of Religion and Spirituality*, No Pagination Specified. https://doi.org/10.1037/rel0000055

Healing the Spiritual Wounds of War | Coming Home Project. http://www.cominghomeproject.net/healing_spiritual_wounds_war

Iraq War Clinician Guide - 2nd Edition - PTSD: National Center for PTSD. http://www.ptsd.va.gov/professional/materials/manuals/iraq-war-clinician-guide.asp

Iraq War Clinician Guide - XI. Traumatic Grief: - iraq_clinician_guide_ch_11.pdf. http://www.ptsd.va.gov/professional/manuals/manual-pdf/iwcg/iraq_clinician_guide_ch_11.pdf

Jinkerson, J. D. (2016). Defining and assessing moral injury: A syndrome perspective. *Traumatology*, *22*(2), 122–130. https://doi.org/10.1037/trm0000069

Kucmin, T., Kucmin, A., Nogalski, A., Sojczuk, S., & Jojczuk, M. (2016). History of trauma and posttraumatic disorders in literature. *Psychiatria Polska, 50*(1), 269–281. https://doi.org/10.12740/PP/43039

Langer, L. L. (1991). *Holocaust Testimonies: The Ruins of Memory*. Yale University Press.

Litz, B. T., Stein, N., Delaney, E., Lebowitz, L., Nash, W. P., Silva, C., & Maguen, S. (2009). Moral injury and moral repair in war veterans: a preliminary model and intervention strategy. *Clinical Psychology Review, 29*(8), 695–706. https://doi.org/10.1016/j.cpr.2009.07.003

Microsoft Word - Moral Injury (1).docx - jpj_moral_injury.pdf. http://www.cjcj. org/uploads /cjcj/documents/jpj_moral_injury.pdf

Moral Injury in Veterans of War - v23n1.pdf. http://www.ptsd.va.gov/professional/newsletters/research-quarterly/v23n1.pdf

Tick, E. (2012). *War and the Soul: Healing Our Nation's Veterans from Post-tramatic Stress Disorder*. Quest Books.

Traumatic Brain Injury. http://www.dcoe.mil/ TraumaticBrainInjury.aspx

Chapter Six:

ADDICTION

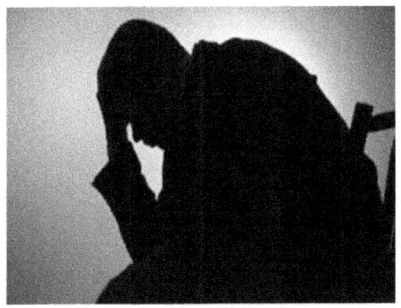

"I have absolutely no pleasure in the stimulants
in which I sometimes so madly indulge.
It has not been in the pursuit of pleasure
that I have periled life and reputation and reason.
It has been the desperate attempt to escape
from torturing memories,
from a sense of insupportable loneliness
and a dread
of some strange impending doom."

Edgar Allan Poe

I begin this chapter with a definition of addiction from the American Society of Addiction Medicine (ASAM). I find it to be broader in scope than the typical delineation, which usually focuses specifically on alcohol or drug addictions from the perspective of an illness model. Furthermore, the authors speak in terms of neuro-circuitry including specified regions of interest in the brain. This comprehensive description follows:

"Addiction is a primary, chronic disease of brain reward, motivation, memory and related circuitry. Addiction affects neurotransmission and interactions within reward structures of the brain . . . such that motivational hierarchies are altered and addictive behaviors, which may or may not include alcohol and other drug use, supplant healthy, self-care related behaviors.

"Addiction also affects neurotransmission and interactions between cortical and hippocampal circuits and brain reward structures, such that the memory of previous exposures to rewards (such as food, sex, alcohol and other drugs) leads to a biological and behavioral response to external cues, in turn triggering craving and/or engagement in addictive behaviors.

"The neurobiology of addiction encompasses more than the neurochemistry of reward. The frontal cortex of the brain and underlying white matter connections between the frontal cortex and circuits of reward, motivation and memory are fundamental in the manifestations of altered impulse control, altered judgment, and the dysfunctional pursuit of rewards . . . seen in addiction--despite cumulative adverse consequences experienced from engagement in substance use and other addictive behaviors. . .

"Frontal lobe morphology, connectivity and functioning are still in the process of maturation during adolescence and young adulthood, and early exposure to substance use is another significant factor in the development of addiction. Many neuroscientists believe that developmental morphology is the basis that makes early-life exposure to substances such an important factor." ("ASAM Definition of Addiction,")

With this comprehensive description in mind, I will provide you with my plan of action for the material presented in this chapter. I begin with an introduction to the brain's pleasure center that is associated with the concept of reward.

Since many people appreciate the amazing world of culturally-related food, as I do, I will use this as a model for the pleasure center to further stimulate your gustatory interests. If you are not a 'foodie,' feel free to substitute imagery of chemicals/drugs in your mind to plug into this model.

The pleasure center includes brain structures that support both cognitive and behavioral responses related to wanting (desire for) and liking (pleasurable experiences). I'd like to avoid turning this chapter into an anatomy lesson and rather, will refer to brain structures that comprise the reward system as primarily found within the cortico-basal ganglia-thalamic loop. The authors of the following 1995 article suggest that:

"The basal ganglia circuitry is also designed so as to modulate in a precise manner the neuronal activity of several brain functional systems, which are involved in the direct control of different aspects of psychomotor behavior. Of utmost importance is the action of the basal ganglia on thalamocortical premotor neurons. It is through these neurons, which can be considered as a sort of final common pathway, that the basal ganglia ultimately influence the complex neuronal computation that goes on at cortical levels."(Parent & Hazrati, 1995)

For those of you interested in further detail pertaining to the neuro-circuitry of the pleasure center, there is ample literature available online for you to explore this topic further. We now move into the tasty world of gustatory experiences. Morton Kringelbach of Oxford and Aarhus Universities describes the effects of food intake as follows.

"A multilevel model of food intake describes the changes over time in: "A) pleasure, B) the levels of hunger, C) satiation/satiety cascade signals, D) origin of signals and signal carriers, E) brain processes, F) behavioural changes including those in the digestive system and G) general modulatory factors. . .

"The multisensory experience of food intake involves all the senses with different routes into the brain; from the distant processing of sight, sound and tactile of food to more proximal smell, taste and tactile (mouth-feel) processing.

"Smell is the most important determinant of the flavour of food and comes to the brain via orthonasal and retronasal pathways, experienced as we breathe in and out, respectively. As demonstrated by the case with coffee, the subjective olfactory experience can feel very different from smelling the coffee in the cup to tasting the coffee in the mouth, which also relies on pure tastants (such as bitter) and mouth feel factors (such as the smoothness of the crema).

"This sensory information about food is coming from receptors in the body, typically the eyes, ears, nose and oral cavity and gets processed in the primary sensory cortices of the brain. . . Importantly, unlike the other senses, olfactory processing is not processed via the thalamus which may explain the hedonic potency of odours. . .

"Neuroscience has started to map the pleasure system in many species. This has been shown to include a number of important regions such as pleasure hotspot regions in subcortical areas of the brain . . . The pleasure system does not act in splendid isolation but is of course embedded within much larger brain networks." (Kringelbach, 2015)

Most drugs of abuse flood the pleasure circuitry with Dopamine, which is a neurotransmitter that regulates movement, emotion, motivation, and feelings of pleasure. When activated normally, the system rewards our natural behaviors. With over-stimulation, euphoric effects are produced that strongly reinforce repetitious drug use behavior. Dopamine enables us to perceive and seek rewards. Persons with low dopamine levels may be prone to sensation seeking behavior.

The focus of discussion will now shift to the incidence of addiction among our active and retired military personnel. More specifically, I will explore the relationships among PTSD, emotional regulatory difficulties and involvement with addictive agents. Among the topics briefly explored within this complex will be eating disorders, online pornography addiction, compulsive gambling, and child pornography and its effect on law enforcement personnel.

This will be followed by an inquiry into the contribution that childhood trauma likely plays in the later emergence of addictive difficulties in life. I will also discuss the issue of Veteran homelessness and its linkage with PTSD and addiction. Instruction in the utilization of RESET-Addiction Therapy will be provided. Finally, comparative case studies will exemplify two varied treatment approaches as they apply to addictive circumstances.

We begin this discourse with a 2016 study that focused on the degree of involvement of our active and retired military personnel in addictive experiences. The authors noted that:

> More than 40% of U.S. military veterans have a lifetime history of alcohol use disorder (AUD). Veterans with a lifetime history of AUD have substantial comorbid psychiatric burden, including elevated rates of suicidal ideation and attempts." (Fuehrlein et al., 2016)

Another 2016 study pertaining to the relationship between post-traumatic stress disorder, problematic alcohol usage and those who have difficulty with regulating emotions is clearly an area of interest. My own perspective is that alcohol, being legally obtained and readily available, becomes a chemical of choice utilized to avoid/suppress/dissociate from the emotion impact of trauma. The authors examining this association noted that:

> Findings revealed that those with trauma and clinically significant PTSD reported greater difficulty with emotion regulation than those who had not been exposed to trauma, which in turn significantly predicted alcohol use. This mediating effect was not found in those

with trauma exposure alone, suggesting an important role for PTSD in this pathway." (Radomski & Read, 2016)

My personal belief is that trauma is frequently at the core of the addictive personality. As a society, we pay a tremendous price for ignoring or ineptly intervening in abusive childhood developmental processes. In this sense, we are a hands-off society, inclined to ignore troubling circumstances with children rather than straightforwardly addressing them. Unfortunately, we 'pay the piper' later through the emergence of socially unacceptable behaviors in those we have so long ignored.

To further complicate the problem, unlike past generations we increasingly immerse ourselves in technology and social media rather than interacting with each other on a personal level. The traditional structures such as the church, community centers, etc., are diminishing in their influence, further adding to isolative tendencies in our communities. In essence, within the context of a culture-rich environment a child thrives. In a deprived or abusive environment, the child's potential becomes limited with negative consequences that later impact or stifle potential.

To further explain my perspective, I'll provide the reader with a 2012 article related to childhood maltreatment and its consequent cortical impact. The investigators inquired into the underlying mechanisms that produce long-lasting impairments in behavioral, cognitive and social functioning.

"A small study was conducted that involved nineteen adolescent volunteers without a history of psychiatric disturbance. However, all of the participants in this group had experienced maltreatment in their childhood years. In contrast, a group consisting of thirteen adolescent volunteers with no history of psychiatric disturbance served as a comparative control group. All volunteers were provided with diffusion tensor imaging (DTI) studies.

"The participants were then followed longitudinally at 6-month intervals for up to 5 years to determine the onset of mood and substance use disorders. . . All of the teens were followed up every six months for an average of three and a half years.

"During that time, the authors found that five of the maltreated children and one control had developed major depression and four of the maltreated children and one control had developed substance use disorders. (Two of the maltreated children had both a drug problem and depression.) This meant that nearly half the maltreated children had either a diagnosable drug problem or depression or both, three times the rate seen in controls. . .

"Using a brain-imaging technique that measures the integrity of the white matter that connects various brain regions, the researchers looked for any differences in the teens' brains when they were first enrolled in the study, before they had developed any psychiatric problems. The scans showed that kids who had been maltreated showed connectivity problems in several brain areas . . . which (are) involved in planning behavior and . . . language processing.

"Another affected region . . . helps connect the brain's emotional processing regions with those involved in more abstract thought, ideally allowing the person to integrate both types of information and to regulate their response to emotional stress." (Huang, Gundapuneedi, & Rao, 2012)

I noticed a 2015 meta-analysis of research covering the period from 1987 to 2014 on the topic of Veteran homelessness. Because one of the core factors associated with this circumstance is adverse childhood experiences, I've included selected material from the article. The authors note that:

"[T]his is the first systematic review to summarize research on risk factors for homelessness among US veterans and to evaluate the evidence for these risk factors. Thirty-one studies published from 1987 to 2014 were divided into 3 categories: more rigorous studies, less rigorous studies, and studies comparing homeless veterans with homeless nonveterans. The strongest and most consistent risk factors were substance use disorders and mental illness, followed by low income and other income-related factors.

"There was some evidence that social isolation, adverse childhood experiences, and past incarceration were also important risk factors. Veterans, especially those who served since the advent of the all-volunteer force, were at greater risk for homelessness than other adults. Homeless veterans were generally older, better educated, and more likely to be male, married/have been married, and to have health insurance coverage than other homeless adults." (Tsai & Rosenheck, 2015)

The issue of homelessness among veterans is mostly qualitative, with few rigorous studies demonstrating causal evidence between risk factors and homelessness. With this in mind, I begin discussion on this topic by referring to a Congressional report submitted by the U.S. Department of Housing and Urban Development entitled: The 2014 Annual Homeless Assessment Report (AHAR included the following material: "on a single night in January 2013 there were 49,993 homeless veterans in the United States. Just under 10% of these veterans were women. Homeless veterans account for 11% of all homeless individuals." ("National Coalition for Homeless Veterans,")

In 2009, the Obama administration committed to ending veteran homelessness by 2015. Although this goal has not been met, veteran homelessness has decreased 33% (National Alliance to End Homelessness, 2015) . . . California has the highest number of homeless veterans, representing 24% of the total population of homeless veterans, followed by Florida (9%), Texas (5%), and New York (5%)." (HUD, 2014)

"Many homeless veterans have mental health problems, alcohol and/or substance abuse issues, and other co-occurring disorders (NCHV,). TBIs were found in 47% of homeless veterans who sought services at a VA hospital.

"America's homeless veterans have served in World War II, the Korean War, the cold war, the Vietnam War, Grenada, Panama, Lebanon, Afghanistan, Iraq, and the military's anti-drug-cultivation efforts in South America; nearly half of all homeless veterans served during the Vietnam era individuals." ("National Coalition for Homeless Veterans,"), ("Homeless_ Veterans_ US.pdf,")

A 2010 article also caught my attention due to its inclusion of the terms 'Drug Memory Reconsolidation' in the title. The authors concluded that:

"[M]emory reconsolidation could potentially be exploited to disrupt, or even erase, aberrant memories that underlie psychiatric disorders, thereby providing a novel therapeutic target. Drug addiction is one such disorder; it is both chronic and relapsing, and one prominent risk factor for a relapse episode is the presentation of environmental cues that have previously been associated with drugs of abuse. . .

"Relapse, the resumption of drug-seeking and drug-taking behaviour following a period of abstinence, can be unconscious, automatic and habitual (and is markedly influenced by the presence of environmental stimuli and contexts that have been paired previously with drug use. These drug-associated conditioned stimuli (CSs), or cues, can induce craving and activate limbic cortico-striatal circuitry in abstinent human addicts. . .

"treatments based upon the disruption of reconsolidation would be predicted to require few, and possibly even a single, treatment with a memory-disrupting drug in order to increase the likelihood of long-lasting abstinence from drugs of abuse. . . treatments need to be developed that can target neurotransmitter systems involved in drug memory reconsolidation . . . without producing unacceptable side-effects in human patients." (Milton & Everitt, 2010)

In fact, a treatment based upon the opportunity to intervene in the reconsolidation process without 'memory-disrupting drugs' currently exists and is referred to as RESET-Addiction. This treatment typically begins with the patient being advised to come in for the session while limiting the addictive agent so that the craving is magnified. A smoker, for example, would not have smoked for some time before the session permitting him/her to more easily tune into the craving.

As discussed in prior chapters and concerning other target circumstances, the BAUD Frequency Knob will be set to resonate with the target which in this case is the craving aspect of the addiction. This is then followed by the Disrupter Knob being adjusted to weaken the targeted circuitry. During the treatment session, the patient/client is asked to focus on the craving for a while but then focus on multiple aspects such as the sensory memory of actually smoking including all of the senses involved.

With earlier discussed conditions such as depression and trauma (PTSD), the instruction related to RESET Therapy has been to 'tune in' to the negative target, adjust the binaural sound to resonate with it and then tune the Disrupter Knob to a point where the emotional aspect began to dissipate.

With addiction, there is a somewhat different approach in that we seek to also *up-regulate* selected neural activity in the pleasure center network while simultaneously down-regulating varied stimuli associated with the addiction experience.

We are able to increase those minimized impulses in us that are not as active as we would like them to be through a neuro-modulatory focus. For example, with emotional trauma, a tendency to pull into a defensive, protective mode rapidly develops. When the fear/anger/etc. switch is reset, growth interest re-emerges leading to an upsurge in social interaction and involvement.

With addiction, the re-emergence of growth tendencies is not quite as simple. Due to the power of urges that develop over the development of the addictive process, extra steps are necessary. Let's take a moment and return to the ASAM definition of addiction that includes the following paragraph:

> Addiction affects neurotransmission and interactions within reward structures of the brain . . . such that motivational hierarchies are altered and addictive behaviors, which may or may not include alcohol and other drug use, supplant healthy, self-care related behaviors. ("ASAM Definition of Addiction,")

Consequently, as we activate the pleasure centers in drug addicts, facilitating them to respond in a normative fashion, we enhance the patient's potential to resist cravings for the chemical of choice. However, because of the strength developed due to the effects of the addictive agent, the cravings had become so strong that we must take the extra step of selectively weakening them.

To accomplish this objective, those triggers associated with the 'high' of the craving stimuli aspect are 'nuked' by the 'healing sound' to facilitate the re-emergence of pleasurable senses that are not associated with the addictive experience. Earlier, I noted that: with over-stimulation, euphoric effects are produced that strongly reinforce repetitious drug use behavior. As also described previously:

> Frontal lobe morphology, connectivity and functioning are still in the process of maturation during adolescence and young adulthood, and early exposure to substance use is another significant factor in the development of addiction. ("ASAM Definition of Addiction,")

Thus, the challenge of establishing 'normalcy' in those utilizing addictive agents earlier in the developmental phases of life becomes even more complex. In these circumstances, increased focus is necessary in diminishing the power of stimuli associated with the addictive urge as well as the pleasure derived from the use of the addictive agent. As an example, the following procedure utilizes the urge to smoke to exemplify the targeting of aspects of the addiction.

He would imagine experiencing the "rush" as the nicotine hit his bloodstream and the 'high' that comes next. He would visualize the smoke curling up before him and the sensation of warmth entering his lungs. After a while, the client is asked to switch to the memory of the satiation or satisfaction felt when he is done with the drug of choice.

In general, the urge-suppressing effects of RESET-Addiction reduces craving for 2 to 3 days before a 'creep-back' effect begins to occur. One might perceive that if the urge returns within hours, the session was likely to have been ineffective indicating the need to again repeat the 'tuning in' process.

The treatment seems to reduce the physiological symptoms of withdrawal typically referred to as urge. If a particularly unpleasant symptom comes up such as nausea, it should become the next target focus either immediately or at the next treatment session.

While targeting the physiological urge to use, the patient will simultaneously engage the neural circuits that connect emotional content to the 'urge.' It is advised that the patient do a specific session focused on neutralizing associated emotional triggers.

As an example, one therapist reported a drug addict who felt the urge to use when he drove past his old dealer's house, leading him to drive miles out of his way to avoid this trigger. Another example would be that of a smoker who felt the urge when in a specific social situation. The emotional trigger might also be feeling the wife's rejection or another painful perception such as recall of a trauma that the addict attempts to cover through addictive arousal.

We now shift focus to the overuse of pornography to a level where it becomes the primary means through which satisfaction of the sexual urge is obtained by the patient. Using the seesaw as an image, imagine that it is tipped totally in one direction. Our therapeutic objective is to simultaneously weaken the powerful (urge) part while strengthening the weak aspect thereby tipping it in the desired direction

With pornography, both desire and reward pathways are sensitized, so they should probably be treated as separate component targets. On some rare occasions, if the Disruptor setting is not set correctly it can inadvertently stimulate a desire to use. Therefore, with the first session, it may be beneficial to "check in" with the patient after a few minutes to make sure the craving is diminishing (or at least, not growing). It would be wise to warn the client that if this should occur, the treatment should be halted and the frequency and disrupter dials should be reset.

With regard to the frequency of sessions, they should be scheduled proactively in order to keep the urge from reappearing. Some therapists have made RESET-Addiction available in their office for a client to self-administer on an as-needed basis as a preventive measure. Others advise purchase of the equipment so that it is available to the patient whenever necessary.

Once a patient has successfully reduced the craving from a treatment session, the therapist should advise that if the craving seems to be returning, place attention and focus back to where it was during the previous session, and remember/hum the resonant sound. I have had several reports that the effect often re-neutralizes the craving.

We will now compare a 'Gold Standard' intervention called Prolonged Exposure Therapy with RESET-Addiction Therapy. The patient in the PET case example presents with all of the features typically associated with the Iraq war experience including: PTSD, TBI, depression and alcohol addiction. A unique aspect of the treatment process involves the utilization of telehealth technology. The details of this case study include the following:

"He is a 22-year-old single, white man, who served 2 tours of duty in Iraq, presented to a Veteran's Administration Medical Center in the southeastern United States. While serving in Iraq, the patient experienced multiple (30) combat fire-fights, witnessed many dead and mutilated bodies, and was seriously wounded twice. . .

"While serving in Iraq, the patient experienced an injury from an improvised explosive device (IED), which led to loss of consciousness, shrapnel impact to his face and neck, a perforated left eardrum, and short-term memory loss. Two months subsequent to this injury, the patient experienced another blast, which led to vertigo, confusion, severe headaches, and tinnitus and loss of hearing for several days.

"The patient lived in a rural area over 100 miles from the nearest Veteran's Administration Medical Center; accordingly, telehealth technology (i.e., videoconferencing) was used. . . [within the context of a] community–based outpatient clinic for 11 weekly, 90-minute sessions conducted over videoconferencing, with a clinical psychologist specialized in treating PTSD. . .

"After the patient's second week of imaginal and in vivo exposure work (session 4), he reported a dramatic drop in intrusive memories and a lessening of the intensity of distress when awoken by nightmares. . . During this time, however, the patient was still experiencing flashbacks, but he reported that the flashbacks were becoming easier to 'break out of.' The patient also reported continued sleep difficulties.

"Despite the fact that no interventions targeted alcohol dependence or depression, the patient also evidenced significant improvement in those areas at session 11. . . a review of the clinical notes indicates that the patient's decrease in substance use coincided to his decrease in distress from intrusions." (Tuerk, Brady, & Grubaugh, 2009)

This case clearly indicates a successful outcome utilizing a novel methodology (video-conferencing) in a systematic manner. Fortunately, the patient was among the one third (as perceived by your present author, based upon studies of efficacy of "Gold Standard" treatments) who respond in a positive manner to an "evidence-based prolonged exposure protocol for PTSD." But what about the two thirds who either respond negatively or not at all? (Hoge et al., 2016)

The following case example is provided as an example of an alternative intervention to Prolonged Exposure Therapy. Jack provided his own first person account with regard to his difficulties with sexual addiction by noting that:

"I first came into contact with RESET Therapy when it was suggested by my counselor, (E. B. – Asheville, N.C.) as a tool to help cope with my sexual addiction cravings. Preceding my first session, I was instructed to recall an emotionally, mentally and physically charged event in my past.

"I choose one such event I possessed that involved an immense amount of shame around an instance in which I paid to have sexual intercourse with a woman. Typically, when the memory would arise, it would persist like a nagging yet powerful force tormenting my thoughts and emotions.

"However, after just one session using RESET, the event went from being a significantly charged memory to a memory remembered from a distance. The memory went from feeling like duct tape wrapped around my consciousness to sand slipping between my fingers.

"I was able to recall the memory from a detached state in which I found incredible relief and a significant decrease in sexual craving. Since that first contact with RESET, my sexual cravings have diminished tenfold, and I've felt a freedom from my sexual addiction that I had not known prior to using the intervention.

"Since my first and only guided RESET Therapy session, my recovery from sex addiction has continued to progress in ways I didn't think were possible. It has been over a month since that first session, and my sexual arousal, particularly of the erotic capacity, has gone from an emotional, impulsivity rating of 7 on a scale from 1 to 10 (high) to a rating of 3 (low end).

"Prior to using RESET, my physical arousal arose impulsively within seconds of visual stimulation or fantasy. Now however, the fantasies and voyeuristic tendencies have become minimal and lost their emotional and energetic hold on me.

"My compulsive sexual behaviors and thoughts have diminished nearly to the point of extinction. When thoughts of a sexual nature do arise, I have been given enough distance from the emotional charge they held in the past to constructively transform that energy in healthy ways."

Two different treatments for addiction were discussed with this patient, with the traditional model requiring eleven ninety-minute treatment sessions. If you will recall, I've taken the position that if insomnia or nightmare/flashbacks are not absent at the conclusion of treatment, the provided intervention is a failure in fully resetting the involved neuronal network back to its normative state. Judged by this criterion, the 'Gold-Standard' treatment was unsuccessful in accom-plishing the designated criteria.

Alternatively, with one RESET-Addiction treatment session, significant and lasting change occurred in the addictive target of concern. My own inclination would have been to provide follow-up sessions to block relapse possibilities. Furthermore, additional remediation of earlier trauma-related material might have strengthened abstinence capacity in this individual.

This RESET-Addiction treated patient did not report sleep disturbance but rather, a pre-occupation with pornography. Because of this, we cannot directly compare the two preceding cases although clearly, changes forthcoming from one hour of neuro-modulation intervention compared to eleven ninety-minute sessions is impressive in its own right.

It was earlier discussed that we can *up-regulate* neural activity in specific brain areas. I noted that through a neuro-modulatory focus, one can selectively strengthen or weaken particular excitatory or suppressed stimuli. I also noted that: as we target activation of the pleasure centers in drug addicts facilitating them to respond in a normative fashion, we enhance the patient's potential to resist cravings for the chemical of choice.

Dr. Frank Lawlis has suggested that the patient think of (activate) joy or pleasure (remembering anything but the addictive problem) and tuning in the Pitch Knob slowly until he/she perceives an *increase* in this sensation. After several minutes of experimentation with the Disruptor Knob, proceeding to tune it until an even *bigger increase* in the positive sensation is experienced.

When the patient feels even more pleasure, the setting can be utilized to enhance visualizing, remembering, sensing, activating a positive affective state. Note: if the Disruptor does not increase the positive affective state, reset it to 0 and use the Pitch Knob only while mentally activating the desired feelings - emotional or physical.

Similar treatment methodology can be utilized with other addictive difficulties such as excessive eating, pathological gambling, excessive video gaming, and for our First Responders, the deleterious effect that child pornography has on police personnel. References that follow will briefly cover the above stated issues by my providing you with pertinent and recent material on the varied topics.

I came upon a 2012 dissertation completed at the University of South Africa that offers an interesting twist regarding child pornography and its effect on law enforcement personnel. Selected members of the South African Police Force must review the material in order to pursue legal action against those that traffic in this filth. The author noted that the:

"[C]onvergence of technology has made access to the Internet faster, easier and cheaper. Criminals, including paedophiles, child abusers and pornography traders make use of this technology to commit criminal offences. Computer Forensic Examiners (CFEs) are members of the Cyber Crime Unit, a professional, specialised unit of the South African Police Service (SAPS) who are responsible for computer forensic examination including the investigation of child pornographic images.

"Analysis of the data . . . clearly showed that all participants were psychologically deeply affected by the constant exposure to child pornography. Based on the themes that were extracted from the conversations that were held with the participants, it was clear that none of the participants were prepared for their first encounter with the material.

"All participants elaborated on the emotions of horror and disgust that they experienced. . . All participants showed negative intra-personal and inter-personal effects. . .

"The CFEs were found to be affected by the culture of the broader Police as well as by the community they serve and are a part of. The relationship the CFE has with his colleagues, family and the community was found to play a role in their experience. The CFEs were deeply affected by the images, and they experienced feelings of distrust toward others that lead to over-protectiveness of their children.

"They also experienced feelings of isolation, where they did not have anyone to share their feelings with. They felt aggressive, angry, frustrated and desperate, and although most of the participants have been working as CFEs for a long time, they do not seem to become desensitised towards the material they are exposed to.

"All participants felt that they had a calling to do the work. They showed a passion for caring for and protecting the innocent and to remove the perpetrators from society. All participants showed an almost desperate need for intervention and debriefing and shared coping skills that they learnt in the process.

"The findings from the interviews with the participants, . . . were found to overlap in many ways. By integrating these findings several symptoms related to traumatic events in general, emerged . . . These symptoms include the following: Desensitising; Trauma and stress; Vicarious traumatization; Compassion fatigue; Burnout; Post-traumatic stress disorder." (Whelpton, 2012)

You might be wondering why I've included this material in the discussion. I had thought about saving it for inclusion in my next book in the PTSD series focusing on First Responders. Alternatively, I thought that the material was too important to hold it back for a prolonged period of time.

Our police, whether they serve in South Africa or the United States deserve to know that they don't have to live with the nightmare of trauma that they have incurred in the line of duty. The same relief can be provided them through the RESET Therapy process as it is applied to the Combat-Veteran with PTSD.

A 2016 study focused on pathological gambling and its association with comorbid disorders, such as anxiety, depression, and drug and alcohol abuse. The authors proposed that:

"Difficulties of emotion regulation may be one of the factors related to the presence of addictive disorders, along with comorbid symptomatology in pathological gamblers. Therefore, the aim of this study was to evaluate the difficulties of emotion regulation, drug and alcohol abuse, and anxious and depressive symptomatology in pathological gamblers, and the mediating role of difficulties of emotion regulation between anxiety and pathological gambling.

"Relative to non-gamblers, pathological gamblers exhibited greater difficulties of emotion regulation, as well as more anxiety, depression, and drug abuse. Moreover, pathological gambling correlated with emotion regulation difficulties, anxiety, depression, and drug abuse.

Besides, emotion regulation difficulties correlated with and predicted pathological gambling, drug and alcohol abuse, and anxious and depressive symptomatology. Finally, emotion regulation difficulties mediated the relationship between anxiety and pathological gambling controlling the effect of age, both when controlling and not controlling for the effect of other abuses." (Jauregui, Estévez, & Urbiola, 2016)

An issue related to our increasing use of technology has been excessive use of video games that may be associated with sleep deprivation, poor job performance and atypical mood disorders. The authors of this 2015 study discussed three active duty service members in the U.S. Marine Corps who were offered mental health evaluation for sleep disturbance and symptoms of blunted affect, low mood, poor concentration, inability to focus, irritability, and drowsiness.

"All three patients reported insomnia as their primary complaint. When asked about online video games and sleep hygiene practices, all three patients reported playing video games from 30 hours to more than 60 hours per week in addition to maintaining a 40-hour or more workweek.

"Our patients endorsed sacrificing sleep to maintain their video gaming schedules without insight into the subsequent sleep deprivation. During the initial interviews, they exhibited blunted affects and depressed moods, but appeared to be activated with enthusiasm and joy when discussing their video gaming with the clinical provider. . .

"Because excessive video gaming is becoming more prevalent worldwide, military mental health providers should ask about video gaming when patients report problems with sleep." (Eickhoff et al., 2015)

Summary

An ASAM definition of addiction was provided that utilizes and incorporates neuroscientific principles as well as recognizes neuro-anatomical locations involved in the addiction process. With this foundation, the reader was next directed to the brain's pleasure center utilizing gustatory descriptors to clarify the role the pleasure center plays in sustaining the addictive process.

Recent information about the incidence of addiction among our active and retired military was provided with note made that 40% of U.S. military veterans have a lifetime history of alcohol use disorder (AUD). The issue of difficulty with regulating emotions takes center stage among many recent studies seeking to clarify who in particular is susceptible to the addictive process.

Within this context, child abuse or neglect during the formative years appears to be one of the primary contributors to the onset of emotional dysregulation. Research is uncovering changes in underlying brain structures consequent to early neglect or abuse. Brain-imaging that measures the brain's white matter revealed connectivity problems in several brain areas of maltreated children.

A systematic review summarizing research on homeless US veterans covering thirty-one studies published from 1987 to 2014 was provided. One of the contributing factors in circumstances of this type is the presence of childhood abuse.

I reiterated my belief that trauma is frequently at the core of the addictive personality. The topic of technology and social media was introduced with associated topics discussed around this issue such as that of gaming addiction and child pornography. To be clear, examples provided in this chapter are illustrative of varied addictive focus.

The chapter is not intended to be a comprehensive review of all possible forms of addiction. The utilization of RESET-Addiction was discussed at length describing how the Frequency and Disruptor Knobs can be tuned to resonate with varied targets such as cravings, withdrawal effects and pleasure.

Two case studies were compared with the first utilizing Prolonged Exposure Therapy (PET) and the second approaching the addictive condition with RESET-Addiction. PET was utilized for 11 weekly, 90-minute sessions. The treating psychologist does not report cessation of alcohol use nor does he refer to complete absence of insomnia and sleep disturbance.

Alternatively, RESET-Addiction treatment appears to be a viable, non-invasive treatment alternative, compared to a traditional form of intervention, that must be explored scientifically. The concept of altered neuronal networks appears to have direct application to addictive disorders potentially leading to remediation and transformation of those struggling with this challenging condition.

Additionally, the reduced time required to obtain sobriety is a major, efficacious first step to reactivating the brain's executive functioning, prefrontal lobe ability. Those who began their addictive process early in life will require training in executive functioning in order to fully develop a full range of cortical potential.

Reference List:

ASAM Definition of Addiction. (2011, April 19). http://www.asam.org/quality-practice/definition-of-addiction

Eickhoff, E., Yung, K., Davis, D. L., Bishop, F., Klam, W. P., & Doan, A. P. (2015). Excessive Video Game Use, Sleep Deprivation, and Poor Work Performance Among U.S. Marines Treated in a Military Mental Health Clinic: A Case Series. *Military Medicine, 180*(7), e839-843. https://doi.org/10.7205/MILMED-D-14-00597

Fuehrlein, B. S., Mota, N., Arias, A. J., Trevisan, L. A., Kachadourian, L. K., Krystal, J. H., … Pietrzak, R. H. (2016). The burden of alcohol use disorders in U.S. Military veterans: results from the national health and resilience in veterans study. *Addiction (Abingdon, England).* https://doi.org/10.1111/add.13423

Hoge, C. W., Yehuda, R., Castro, C. A., McFarlane, A. C., Vermetten, E., Jetly, R., … Rothbaum,

B. O. (2016). Unintended Consequences of Changing the Definition of Posttraumatic Stress Disorder in DSM-5: Critique and Call for Action. *JAMA Psychiatry*, *73*(7), 750–752. https://doi.org/10.1001/jamapsychiatry.2016.0647

Homeless_Veterans_US.pdf. https://www.ebscohost.com/assets-sample-content/Homeless_Veterans_US.pdf

Huang, H., Gundapuneedi, T., & Rao, U. (2012). White matter disruptions in adolescents exposed to childhood maltreatment and vulnerability to psychopathology. *Neuropsychopharmacology: Official Publication of the American College of Neuropsychopharmacology*, *37*(12), 2693–2701. https://doi.org/10.1038/npp.2012.133

Jauregui, P., Estévez, A., & Urbiola, I. (2016). Pathological Gambling and Associated Drug and Alcohol Abuse, Emotion Regulation, and Anxious-Depressive Symptomatology. *Journal of Behavioral Addictions*, *5*(2), 251–260. https://doi.org/10.1556/2006.5.2016.038

Kringelbach, M. L. (2015). The pleasure of food: underlying brain mechanisms of eating and other pleasures. *Flavour*, *4*, 20. https://doi.org/10.1186/s13411-014-0029-2

Milton, A. L., & Everitt, B. J. (2010). The psychological and neurochemical mechanisms of drug memory reconsolidation: implications for the treatment of addiction. *European Journal of Neuroscience, 31*(12), 2308–2319. https://doi.org/10.1111/j.1460-9568.2010.07249.x

National Coalition for Homeless Veterans. http://nchv.org/index.php/news/media/background_and_statistics

Parent, A., & Hazrati, L.-N. (1995). Functional anatomy of the basal ganglia. I. The cortico-basal ganglia-thalamo-cortical loop. *Brain Research Reviews, 20*(1), 91–127. https://doi.org/10.1016/0165-0173(94)00007-C

Radomski, S. A., & Read, J. P. (2016). Mechanistic role of emotion regulation in the PTSD and alcohol association. *Traumatology, 22*(2), 113–121. https://doi.org/10.1037/trm0000068

Tsai, J., & Rosenheck, R. A. (2015). Risk Factors for Homelessness Among US Veterans. *Epidemiologic Reviews, 37,* 177–195. https://doi.org/10.1093/epirev/mxu004

Tuerk, P., Brady, K. T., & Grubaugh, A. L. (2009). Clinical Case Discussion: Combat PTSD and Substance Use Disorders: *Journal of Addiction Medicine, 3*(4), 189–193. https://doi.org/10.1097/ADM.0b013e3181a9d276

Whelpton, J. (2012). The psychological effects experienced by computer forensic examiners working with child pornography. Retrieved from http://uir.unisa.ac.za/handle/10500/6217

Chapter Seven:

COMPLEX PTSD

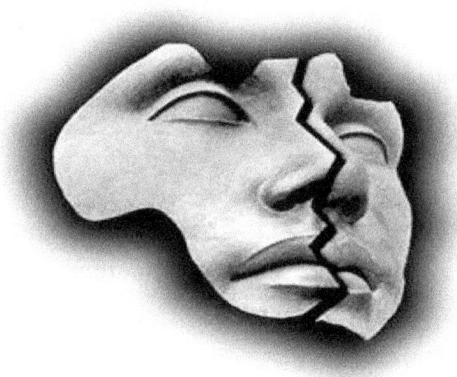

"Unlike simple stress, trauma changes your view of your life and yourself. It shatters your most basic assumptions about yourself and your world — "Life is good," "I'm safe," "People are kind," "I can trust others," "The future is likely to be good" — and replaces them with feelings like "The world is dangerous," "I can't win," "I can't trust other people," or "There's no hope."

Mark Goulston, Post-Traumatic Stress Disorder For Dummies

There is little question in my mind that treating someone with Complex PTSD is a challenging, at times, harrowing task. Attempting to establish the "trust relationship" purported to be essential in traditional therapy can become an insurmountable challenge in and of itself with this type of patient. One problem has been that before the notion of developmental trauma surfaced, varied misdiagnoses defined the patient such as Borderline Personality Disorder, Multiple Personality Disorder, etc.

Let's take a look at where the term, Complex PTSD (CPTSD) came into being formally. It was described first in 1992 and later by the same author in 1997 as a post-trauma syndrome characterized by problems in the domains of:

> interpersonal relationships, somatization, affect regulation, dissociation, and sense of self." (Judith Lewis Herman, 1992), (Judith Lewis Herman, 1997a)

A further clarification took place in 2013 when three CPTSD symptom clusters were proposed including:

> affect dysregulation, negative self-concept, and interpersonal disturbances.

Maercker et al. also specified that:

the affect dysregulation criterion would include emotional reactivity, dissociation, anger, aggression, and emotional numbing. Negative self-concept would be defined by negative beliefs about the core value of the self along with feelings of guilt and shame. Interpersonal disturbances would include avoidance of relationships, estrangement, and lack of emotional intimacy in relationships." (Maercker et al., 2013)

"The prior concepts, refined over a number of years, began to solidify the distinctiveness of those that share these tendencies. Now couple this with a historical institutional tendency to deny what earlier was called "battle fatigue" up until the 1980's and now it is called Post-Traumatic Stress Disorder. Those afflicted with this condition adds up to quite a few people, estimated to be over 200,000 from our Vietnam Veterans alone." ("Findings from the National Vietnam Veterans' Readjustment Study - PTSD,")

A study of the aforementioned cluster of symptoms was conducted in 2015 to provide:

"empirical examination and scientific vetting prior to the publication of *ICD-11* because adopting an unvalidated diagnosis has potential to negatively impact scientific advances and clinical care of trauma survivors worldwide.

"Participants in the community sample were 3,756 adults recruited from an online probability-based panel maintained by Survey Sampling International. . . Approximately half (52%) of the sample was female.

". . . Participants reported exposure to a wide range of traumatic events including being a victim of physical or sexual assault (53.1%), death of a family member or close friend due to an accident, violence, or disaster (51.8%), natural disaster (50.5%), accident/fire (48.3%), witnessing a physical or sexual assault (33.2%), threat or injury to a family member or close friend due to violence/accident /disaster (32.4%), and witnessing a dead body unexpectedly (22.6%).

"The second sample included . . . 323 (who) completed the study and were included . . . This sample was 61% male with a mean age of 44 (range: 23 – 85); 80% self-identified as white. . . A majority (75%) had served in OEF/OIF. In addition, 15% served in the Vietnam War era, 4% during the Operation Desert Storm era, and 1% served in the Korean War or World War II eras.

"The prevalence of current CPTSD in the community and veteran samples was 0.6% and 13.0%, respectively. Wolf et. al, suggested that one-fourth of those in the community sample and just under one-half of the veterans with *ICD-11* PTSD also met criteria for CPTSD." (Wolf et al., 2015)

If the above results are truly representative of the Veteran and civilian communities, most of those with the condition go untreated. Extrapolating from the above findings, 50% of Veterans with PTSD are likely to have a complex aspect of the condition.

The US Department of Veterans Affairs, National Center for PTSD, advises that an individual who experienced a prolonged period (months to years) of chronic victimization and total control by another may also experience the following difficulties:

"Emotional Regulation: May include persistent sadness, suicidal thoughts, explosive anger, or inhibited anger.

"Consciousness: Includes forgetting traumatic events, reliving traumatic events, or having episodes in which one feels detached from one's mental processes or body (dissociation).

"Self-Perception: May include helplessness, shame, guilt, stigma, and a sense of being completely different from other human beings.

"Distorted Perceptions of the Perpetrator: Examples include attributing total power to the perpetrator, becoming preoccupied with the relationship to the perpetrator, or preoccupied with revenge.

"Relations with Others. Examples include isolation, distrust, or a repeated search for a rescuer. One's System of Meanings. May include a loss of sustaining faith or a sense of hopelessness and despair." (Complex PTSD - PTSD,)

Psychiatrist Judith Lewis Herman, among other things, has focused throughout her career on the understanding and treatment of traumatic stress. She is a Professor of Clinical Psychiatry at Harvard University Medical School and served as the Director of Training at the Victims of Violence Program in the Department of Psychiatry. In her 1997 book on Trauma and Recovery, she suggested that:

> "standard evidence-based treatments for PTSD are effective for treating PTSD that occurs following chronic trauma. At the same time, treating Complex PTSD often involves addressing interpersonal difficulties and the specific symptoms mentioned above."

At that time (1997) how little did we know that talk or repeatedly exposing someone to traumatic recall were basically ineffective tools. Though I disagree with the above statement, I am, at least, in partial agreement with the following perspective. I have come to understand that 'healing' occurs within the internal brain network as opposed to relationships with others. The following material was taken from the same book:

recovery from Complex PTSD requires restoration of control and power for the traumatized person. Survivors can become empowered by healing relationships which create safety, allow for remembrance and mourning, and promote reconnection with everyday life. (Judith Lewis Herman, 1997b)

Building on the above perspective, Kolb et al., suggest that trauma victims will fail to cope adequately with their problems until they have attained a sense of security in their bodies.

In losing control over their bodily functions they are not the competent people they were before. (Wilson, 2014)

Herman, et al., noted further that:

interfamilial abuse must certainly be included among the most severe traumas encountered by human beings. (J. L. Herman, Perry, & van der Kolk, 1989)

This recognition opens up the boundaries between the current concept of PTSD and what we have called 'the trauma spectrum'. Other post-traumatic disorders ranging from those that result from brief traumatic exposure at an early age, such as phobias and panic, to Borderline Personality Disorder and Multiple Personality Disorder which are usually associated with chronic interfamilial abuse. (B. A. van der Kolk, 1988)

A 2006 study explored how cognitive-behavioral therapy affected a range of outcomes in a sample of urban women with comorbid substance use disorders and PTSD.

"Results show that a majority of participants reported repeated experiences of interpersonal abuse with exposure to trauma beginning at a relatively early age. In addition to PTSD and substance use disorders, a significant portion of participants also met criteria for having an affective disorder.

"Severity of depression and dissociative symptoms was high, as were rates of poly-substance abuse, impulsivity, somatic complaints, and interpersonal problems. After three months, participants in the cognitive-behavioral therapy group had significant reductions in PTSD and alcohol use disorder symptoms.

"A trend was found toward a decrease in drug use disorder symptoms, although it did not reach significance. No significant differences existed between groups on depression, dissociation, and social and sexual functioning outcomes.

"These findings demonstrate that although short-term cognitive-behavioral interventions may decrease some symptom clusters, other problems associated with complex trauma may be less amenable to this type of treatment." (Cohen & Hien, 2006)

Trauma training was offered by Bessel van der Kolk, Ph.D., through the International Society for Traumatic Stress Studies (ISTSS) in a course entitled, "Treating Trauma: Helping the Entire Human Organism Feel Safe and Live in the Present." The trainer proposed that:

"Trauma affects the entire human organism, which gets stuck in neurobiological, immunological and relational survival modes.

"Neuroscience research shows that the brain regions most affected by trauma are involved in attention and perception, biasing the organism into perceiving threat and annihilation. These subcortical processes are independent from conscious appraisal or conscious control.

"This presentation will focus on evidence based treatments that address basic issues of safety, threat appraisal and embodied awareness, illustrated by EMDR, meditation, yoga, theater, martial arts and sensory integration." (B. van der Kolk 2011)

Finally, an article published by Julian Ford entitled, "Recovering from (complex) PTSD by regaining self-regulation." is included within the context of the current discussion. The author suggests that:

the key to recovery (from PTSD) is not rocket science. Survival threats can cause the brain to be hijacked by its own alarm system (link is external), so the key is to re-set that alarm system so it's no longer in survival mode. (PTSD Becomes (More) Complex in the DSM-5: Part II | Psychology Today,)

In sorting through the above perspectives, I propose using an example of turning a light switch on and off. In fact, part of the title of our first published paper is called, 'Resetting the Fear Switch in PTSD'. As discussed in this article, I proposed that the mechanism of action of RESET is to disrupt the reconsolidation of problematic memory circuits within the limbic system of the brain through the use of sound stimulation. ("Resetting the Fear Switch in PTSD,")

While many current treatments may refer to their effects as involving reconsolidation, they do not clarify the specific mechanism of action in their process. Going back to the example, if I were to repeatedly tell the light switch to turn off, what do you think would happen?

How is the evidence-based treatment, referred to by varied researchers, effective when they are not altering the neuronal network that continues to mediate the trauma effects? Perhaps with enough talk therapy the light switch gradually dims but my clinical experience has been that this doesn't fully and completely turn it off.

I would be inclined to agree with Kolb et al., that trauma victims cope inadequately at least partially due to a sense of insecurity in their bodies. (Kolb & Mutalipassi, 1982) In my mind, I absolutely agree with Herman, Perry and van der Kolk's perspective that, "interfamilial abuse must certainly be included among the most severe traumas encountered by human beings." The remediation methods they propose are in the right direction, but likely produce a gradual rather than a complete shift in limbic activity over time.

A 2015 article reported an investigation of whether a "stabilization phase" was necessary within the treatment of CPTSD. This term is defined as:

"teaching self-regulation strategies . . . to ensure that an individual would be better able to tolerate trauma-focused treatment. The purpose of this paper is to critically evaluate the research underlying these treatment guidelines for cPTSD, and to specifically address the question as to whether a phase-based approach is needed.

"As reviewed in this paper, the research supporting the need for phase-based treatment for individuals with cPTSD is methodologic-ally limited. Further, there is no rigorous research to support the views that: (1) a phase-based approach is necessary for positive treatment outcomes for adults with cPTSD, (2) front-line trauma-focused treatments have unacceptable risks or that adults with cPTSD do not respond to them, and (3) adults with cPTSD profit significantly more from trauma-focused treatments when preceded by a stabilization phase.

"The current treatment guidelines for cPTSD may therefore be too conservative, risking that patients are denied or delayed in receiving conventional evidence-based treatments from which they might profit." (De Jongh et al., 2016)

Further challenges to the proscribed way of treating Complex PTSD include the following:

"Evidence of efficacy in studies of post-traumatic conditions is largely derived from studies in which variables are kept to a minimum. Extrapolation of treatments from uncomplicated disorders to complex conditions may therefore be called evidence-based without being evidenced.

"Complex conditions with polysymptomatic presentations and extensive comorbidity are being denied proper evaluation, and patients most severely traumatized from the early stages of their development are not provided with rigorously evaluated psychotherapies because they are more difficult to study in the manner approved by research protocols.

"Such evidence as there is suggests that the simple extension of treatments for uncomplicated disorders is seriously inadequate. This has significant implications for health services responsible for the provision of the most efficacious treatments to those whose disorders arise from severe trauma, often very early in their life." (Corrigan & Hull, 2015)

The following case study in which RESET Therapy was used along with traditional talk therapy is provided to illustrate efficacy in a complicated case that included developmental abuse factors. The patient did not receive a "stabilization phase" but rather, was progressively guided to address his complex inner world of darkness and fear through successfully transforming trauma related material into understanding, insight and growth.

The case is provided also to clarify the treatment process from the patient's perspective. The talk therapy aspect was initiated only after insight emerged resulting from Paul's emotional releasing of pent up repressed affect. The patient detailed his traumatic developmental history as well as his response to the treatment intervention. He did this in a revealing and honest manner as he encountered challenges that have troubled him throughout the course of his lifetime.

What is most encouraging from this non-traditional treatment experience is the normalization that he has been able to attain in a relatively brief period and how this became translated into self-enhancing steps that he was finally able to implement.

Paul was raised within a badly damaged family. Therapists speak of a "weak core personality" in cases such as this. While RESET Therapy is still remarkably successful with PTSD, in complex cases it must be provided in an ongoing series of sessions with a greater level of support than required in non-complex cases.

My treatment relationship with Paul was further complicated because we lived in different locations. Because of this, we primarily used long-distance communication conducted through email and phone. We were able to do this successfully since he had a BAUD as well as local therapeutic support available to him. Might this be a hint of things to come given that we are now fully in the world of ever-changing technology?

'Paul's Story'

"I had a difficult childhood including troubled memories of living in a small three story house with my step-sister and two younger brothers. My mother was separated from my father most of the time that we lived there. Mother was not able to cope with four children, no husband and little financial support. She was born in Russia in 1917 and my understanding is that she had near death experiences during the Bolshevik regime.

"Mom told me that when she was two or three years old, the Bolshevik's were rounding up Jewish people to kill them. She and her family escaped while hiding in a barn. Eventually, her eldest brother helped the family escape to Cuba and then to immigrate to the USA. Mom was terrified of her oldest brother and told stories about how she literally peed in her pants when he would exhibit anger toward her.

"Mom admitted to me and my brothers when we were older that she hated us three boys because to her, we represented our father. She said that she resented him for coercing her to have children and then leaving her alone to raise us. When mom would break down and cry she would say, 'I can't take it anymore, I can't handle this'"

"As an adult I came to believe the same. When I got stressed I learned to give up in frustration and believed that I might die because I could not take it anymore – just like my mom.

"As I got older, about seven to ten, Mom made me responsible for my two younger brothers. I frequently got blamed for everything that went wrong being blamed for what they did or didn't do. My cleaning was never good enough and I was never good enough! Mom constantly used me to release all her anger and hate. I was frequently cursed at, hit at, berated, and screamed at for many years.

"I remember being terrified when she tied me to the boiler in the basement. It was dark and I was very afraid that I would die alone and no one would help me. This started my worst fear that has been with me all my life: that of being frightened to death to be alone. I thought that in that basement I would die and no one would help me. I eventually imagined I was dead and that way she couldn't hurt me anymore.

"Her hurtful words became part of me. The constant berating, cursing and physical abuse caused me to develop a defensive physical posture resulting in my having much difficulty trusting or confiding in myself or others. I learned not to show my emotions like to cry or that I was sad or hurt. I had come to fear the future and frequently projected failure, death, injury, loss. The minute I had something to schedule I would worry: how will I get there; what will I say; will people reject me or insult me or put me down. Fear of rejection and fear of failure became part of my normal thought process.

"From 11 to 17, we relocated to Florida with both my mother and father who later rejoined the family. They got back together and me and my two brothers experienced less anger from mom as she now had some support from my father. Dad had PTSD from WWII and was depressed a lot and quiet when he got home from work. Mostly he would be found curled up on the couch in pain or depressed over things he wouldn't discuss.

"I enlisted in the Marine Corps at the age of 17 over forty-eight years ago. My Marine Corps boot camp training at Parris Island, South Carolina was very stressful, difficult, and traumatic for me. The drill instructors scared all of us so I learned to keep my mouth shut, to listen, and to follow orders like I did with mom. There was a time I was caught talking to another marine recruit in the latrine without permission. The drill instructor became very agitated and choked me for disobeying the rules, really scaring me.

"This was the beginning of a series of deep emotional scars that left a permanent mark deep inside of me. After advanced training I was assigned to a marine regiment in Vietnam that was later known as the Dying Nine. I learned that my battalion was singled out for destruction by the enemy. Our foes called us the Walking Dead. Fortunately, I did not know at the time that the casualty rate for my unit was about 80% killed or wounded.

"I was assigned to the 1st Battalion, 9th Marines - Third Marine Division. My assignment in Vietnam in March of 1968 was at the Khe Sahn combat base around the end of the Tet offensive. [bad place, bad time]

"Instantly I learned how to survive as I became a constant target for the enemy along with my fellow Marines. Much of my anxiety, fear, and hypervigilance came from trying to stay alive while dodging incoming rockets, mortars, and bullets from enemy snipers.

"We were attacked daily with rockets, mortars and bullets from the North Vietnamese Army (NVA). Always there were casualties resulting in dead or wounded Marines. We rarely encountered the enemy face to face as they mostly hid from our view and fired at us from a distance.

"On June 18, 1968, my unit was on patrol. We were resting after reaching the location we were assigned to in Quang Tri Province. An NVA soldier appeared at the edge of the bomb crater I was in and I became startled as he was only about 30 to 40 feet from me.

"When I saw him I immediately stood up and faced him with my M16 rifle in hand. He fired his AK47 assault rifle and a bullet hit my wrist causing my M16 to drop. I immediately crawled to the back of the bomb crater to take protection in the high elephant grass and I crouched down waiting in fear that the enemy would find me helpless. Fortunately, another marine came to my assistance and we crawled over to a shallow depression where we found a corpsman.

"Another wounded marine and I waited there until the firefight was over. I was then transported to a first aid station in Vietnam and then transferred to Japan. Eventually I arrived at Key West Naval Hospital in July of 1968 where I was treated for a shattered wrist and gangrene.

"It took four months of mega doses of antibiotics to take care of the infection. Narcotics were administered daily to kill the pain but they didn't numb me enough to suppress the cries of pain and anguish around the clock from other wounded soldiers.

"I was medically and honorably discharged in February, 1969, from Jacksonville Naval Air Station. Over the next 40 years my mental state got progressively worse due to untreated and severe chronic combat-related PTSD. I turned off all of my emotions in combat except anger and fear with this continuing non-stop after I got out of the military.

"I was in denial that I had PTSD, but was aware that I had anger problems. I tried talk therapy with psychologists for much of those 40 years but that didn't bring relief to my PTSD symptoms. One time I went into a rage and pushed my wife saying, *'stop yelling because you are going to alert the enemy.'*

"Eventually in 2009 the emotional and physical stress elevated to a point where I was having daily panic attacks, homicidal and suicidal ideations, hyper-vigilance, rages, startle response, fears, nightmares, depression and anxiety. I also had chronic neck and low back pain and difficulty with routine everyday activities of daily living.

"Unfortunately, over the last 40 years, traditional treatment such as drug medications and talk therapy have not helped my PTSD symptoms. When I'm triggered, I need to go out somewhere, like I had to escape from the house when I was a child and then come back home to the site of the trauma. I am afraid when I have to leave the house to go on a routine errand or appointment I will not return alive.

"I'm afraid thinking that I may die like in Vietnam prior to going out on another deadly patrol. The company commander would shout out: *OK men,*

'Saddle up! – I thought, I'm going out again on another suicide patrol not knowing if I will return alive. I always thought I would get killed or wounded, just didn't know when.'

"After many years of traditional therapy for my PTSD related symptoms I finally found a therapy that works. I now have a sense of peace and well-being I never had previously. I am better able to cope with everyday routine problems and life issues without constant anxiety and panic attacks. I also found a way to resolve the deep depression that has been with me since Vietnam in 1968. I use both logic and emotion more routinely and can think more quickly. I come up with ideas and express myself more spontaneously.

"My fight or flight switch is turned off and I do not feel the constant adrenalin/cortisol rush from anxiety and fear. I am better able to focus on a single task without intrusive thoughts and dissociation: something that was very prevalent on a daily basis. I feel more relaxed and am able to make decisions based on what is best for me instead of people pleasing.

"I am in the process of deprogramming from the part of my Marine Corps training that is harmful to me in my everyday life. I now know I am not a constant danger to myself and others due to my explosive rage that has been with me all these years.

"In fact, it's significantly diminished! I have a better relationship with my wife and with myself. I sleep better and am not constantly problem solving and obsessing about what to do and how to do it."

****

The following e-mail notes were selected in order to share with you the unfolding therapeutic process that Paul experienced, sometimes on a day to day basis. We met face to face on only one occasion where I adjusted the sound to resonate with his selected trauma. I've included notes that display Paul's emerging awareness of his changing status as well as the positive steps he has taken to function in a world that he has previously been alienated from.

I have not significantly changed the substance of his correspondence with the exception of removing identifying material. My specific e-mail replies to Paul are underlined to provide you with my reactions, directives, etc., in reply to his progress reports. At first, Paul responded on an almost daily basis revealing his strong need and desire for guidance and acceptance.

Ironically, the distance and lack of personal intimacy that is typically developed within the face to face therapeutic experience likely permitted Paul to truly develop a deep and full relationship with me. In retrospect, this seemed to be a good alternative to his going through a difficult transference relationship to get to a point of mutual trust.

Meaningful aspects of his correspondence are included so that you may be an inside observer to the hurdles Paul faced. In addition, you share the tremendous courage he evidenced in pushing through a life time of barriers that blocked him from fully transforming into the person he was truly meant to be.

****

Paul - 3/05/14 "I used the same settings Dr. George found for me when we met and let all of the feelings flow into the sound. The first five to ten minutes, I allowed the feelings within me to surface and saw flashes of anger and fear with my mother, boot camp, Vietnam. Then the last ten minutes or so, the anger and rages and everything subsided and all I could see, hear or feel was the annoying buzzing of the sound. On a scale of 1-10, I felt like I was a zero, quite amazing!"

"Paul, it looks like your setting is good for the anxiety targets. Let me suggest that you use RESET selectively now when the strong feelings come up, particularly with the PTSD triggers.

Paul - 3/7/14 – "I woke up with typical fears like I need women to protect me and looking for my sister to protect me. Later in the afternoon, after a nap, I was in a foul mood and started having the same feeling towards my wife that I had toward mom for locking me up in the basement tied to the boiler and left all alone. I did a treatment with my anger level about an 8 with it going to 1 to 2 when done. I also had back pain at a 7 level on the 10-point pain scale. After treatment my back pain was about a 1. Afterwards, I felt good for the rest of the evening."

Paul - 3/12/14 "Interesting day – woke up and did a treatment right away. I noticed a pattern of awakening with the traumatic memories and accompanying thought processes [a REM sleep process?]. It feels like someone is looking to get at me to kill me or try to harm me. Survival mode thinking still seems normal to me. Not every day is like this but now that I am doing these treatments there is a change in my intensity level."

Paul - 3/13/14 "I did a treatment and wow, it turned out to be mostly about Viet Nam. It was when I was terrified about going out on patrols and not knowing if we were going to die that moment or not. I was able to eventually feel accepting of my traumatic experience. I think that RESET has been reducing my PTSD and now my brain is able to understand and learn new concepts, unlike my survival brain on PTSD."

Paul - 3/14/14 – "I have identified two core issues that are of importance to me. With the first: I have to get out of my house in order to feel and be safe. With the second: I need to have people validate me as being ok, real, worthy and loved. I woke up this morning anxious, thinking I can't wait to leave the house so I can see people."

"Paul, I'm following your notes closely and notice that objectivity is beginning to evidence itself in your reports. This confirms for me that you're really putting yourself fully into the process. Thus, I'd like to take you to the next level in your exploration using RESET Therapy.

"You will be finding that there are different brain circuits through your focusing on them. The first of course is the anxiety/trauma protocol. In essence, you are to become the fear/anxiety throughout the 15/20 minutes of treatment. This is frightening but it is the path to take to fully free you from this aspect of your complex PTSD. Thus, rather than running from the house, you are to stay there & nuke the fear!"

Paul - 3/16/14 "This morning I focused on fully experiencing the fear as you advised. I targeted the feelings in my shoulders and neck and felt it in my body. Eventually thoughts and images arose of the DI in boot camp saying, 'don't look at me and don't talk unless you're given permission.' I did my best to feel and become part of that experience. When it diminished, the next image was of my mother expressing that I should not be seen or heard and to shut up. I went into that experience as fully as I could, seeing it and feeling the fear all over my upper body.

"At first it was difficult not to run from it but I decided not to rush it and to take my time. Eventually I found myself verbalizing it saying out loud, 'I can't talk or you may kill me.' It may have been from childhood or Vietnam or both. Verbalizing it helped me to clarify the specific fear. I noted the settings for future use and noted that today's session was longer than previous ones lasting about 25 minutes. Later in the morning, I noticed some other trauma issues and noted them for my next session."

"Paul, you'll notice that as the trauma poison leaves you, other targets will surface almost in a cue like fashion. After a while, your mind will put them in the hopper instinctively.

"As you develop trust in the process, the core aspects of who you truly are will solidify. You're doing well with becoming more specific with RESET Therapy tuning."

Paul - 4/03/14 "I am changing my attitudes and belief system toward a more positive one. Now, I only use RESET when it is needed. I know that it really works and I'm getting a better awareness and feel for when to use it. The first problem I recognize is my tendency to deny that I have a problem to myself.

"After I admit that I am anxious, I have come to trust that the treatment will help. It really takes time for me to trust anything. It's like peeling off onion layers. When I address a current situation, it seems to connect with and clear up the original cause from the past. Then the next day something that was deeply suppressed in my mind comes up."

"Paul, I'd like to discuss one of your core difficulties which is: 'I have to get out of my house in order to feel and be safe.' Now I believe that your progress suggests that it is time to take this one on. To do it, you must face the fear head-on by staying in the house till it is resolved. Of course, use the RESET-Anxiety setting for this one."

Paul - 4/09/14 "As soon as I saw your e-mail, I took a different approach to RESET. Rather than going into my bedroom to do a RESET intervention, I stayed out in the common living areas and decided to do RESET when I felt the need. I did a RESET without limiting the time I needed to completely resolve the ongoing delusion/flashback.

"I had very positive results so far this weekend with the new concept. I can stay right here and face whatever it is, right in the middle of my real area of stress. I can be around live people and be okay. I appreciate your support and will call if I need to."

"Paul, insight is present in your comments. This is clearly a sign that you are breaking through the instinctive survival reactions and using more advanced processing abilities to figure out what is triggering you. You are reaching your goal."

****

I end the month-and-a-half of comments and responses here as you are certainly aware by now that this is an ongoing therapeutic process. This becomes a much more traditional therapy interchange than the quick results reported in non-complex PTSD cases.

Hopefully, you've also noticed that Paul is now firmly in the world of reality rather than in the delusional mode he was in previously. He is rebuilding his sense of self-esteem, brick by brick. I believe that his addictive difficulties have been stabilized, his marriage has a chance and his hope for the future finally has a firm foundation.

I continue to follow Paul although he rarely needs advice or support now. I consider this to be the best type of compliment I could possibly receive!

Summary

Complex PTSD is considered to be a condition that is a consequence of chronic or long-term exposure to emotional trauma. Within this context, the victim of the abuse has: little or no control or power; has little or no hope of escape; experiences negative developmental effects regarding the emerging self-concept.

The diagnostic identification in DSM-5 remains controversial. In the stressor-related disorders section, the authors write:

> It is clear, however, that many individuals who have been exposed to a traumatic or stressful event exhibit a phenotype in which, rather than anxiety- or fear-based symptoms, the most prominent clinical characteristics are anhedonic and dysphoric symptoms, externalizing angry and aggressive symptoms, or dissociative symptoms. . .

We must conclude, therefore, that DSM-5 has hinted at symptoms of complex PTSD, but in the end has left them out of the manual. DSM-5 continues to opt for a universal reaction to stress, as presented in the diagnostic criteria." ("PTSD in DSM-5," 2015)

The topic of Complex PTSD emerged in the early 90's with refinements of the definition continuing to the present time. A number of symptom clusters have been suggested in an attempt to differentiate this complex entity from the established criteria necessary for the diagnosis of PTSD. These clusters included the following components: affect dysregulation, negative self-concept, and interpersonal disturbances.

A 2015 study by Wolf et. al., that included a community-based sample revealed high levels of exposure to a wide range of traumatic events. A second sample targeted Veterans of whom the majority had served in OEF/OIF. As noted, it was postulated that ¼ of the community-based sample and close to ½ of the Veteran group met criteria for CPTSD.

Commonalities and differences between PTSD and CPTSD were discussed. Attributes of the cluster groupings were expanded upon. Dr. Herman's perspective related to the treatment of Complex PTSD was provided. As you would suspect by now, I partially agree and partially disagree with her perspective.

I have found standard evidence-based treatments for PTSD and CPTSD to be ineffective in fully and totally remediating the symptoms of both conditions. In my mind, the Kolb et al. perspective is right on! The challenge is how to make this happen in an expeditious way.

Dr. van der Kolk and colleagues' concept of "trauma spectrum" was discussed. Results of a 2006 study were provided with a conclusion that suggested that:

> short-term cognitive-behavioral interventions may decrease some symptom clusters, other problems associated with complex trauma may be less amenable to this type of treatment.

I addressed the question of whether a "stabilization phase" was necessary, weighing in on the side of viewing this as an unnecessary hurdle. The phase-related aspect of the treatment that you read about involves my patient removing, layer by layer, the effects of prolonged developmental and combat related trauma in a systematic manner over the period of close to four months. This was accomplished with occasional e-mail or telephone support.

Finally, Dr. Ford's perspective that "recovery (from PTSD) is not rocket science" served as a perfect segue to the RESET Therapy case presentation where the "alarm system" was systematically and progressively reset. Our Veteran revealed a multigenerational history of trauma, detailing his mother's recollection of her childhood Russian experience as well as his father's war-incurred PTSD.

Clearly, his earlier years were difficult with his mother projecting her distain for men onto him and his younger brothers. The seed of his dissociative tendencies are clearly evident in his reported incidents such as being "tied to a boiler in a darkened basement." One would question, based solely upon his early experiences, whether remediation was even possible.

Paul incorporated his negative projections, becoming one with each of them. In essence, every cell in his body was switched to a defensive, protective mode. This was compounded by his military involvement in the nightmare of combat in Vietnam. Upon his release from service, his undiagnosed PTSD and Complex PTSD raged on. Over the course of 40 years, traditional treatment failed him.

Paul's report of his RESET Therapy experience is illustrative of what I've heard from so many of my patients. What remains is to validate the intervention through comprehensive and standardized research. Soon this will happen with a recent Institutional Review Board (IRB) approval of a study using RESET Therapy with 36-combat Veterans in the Gulf Coast region of Florida. This is our first major step in brings this amazing treatment to public awareness.

Reference List:

Cohen, L. R., & Hien, D. A. (2006). Treatment Outcomes for Women With Substance Abuse and PTSD Who Have Experienced Complex Trauma. *Psychiatric Services (Washington, D.C.)*, *57*(1), 100–106. https://doi.org /10.1176/appi.ps.57.1.100

Complex PTSD - PTSD: National Center for PTSD. http://www.ptsd.va.gov/professional/PTSD-overview/complex-ptsd.asp

Corrigan, F. M., & Hull, A. M. (2015). Neglect of the complex: why psychotherapy for post-traumatic clinical presentations is often ineffective. *BJPsych Bull*, *39*(2), 86–89. https://doi.org/10.1192/pb.bp.114. 046995

De Jongh, A., Resick, P. A., Zoellner, L. A., van Minnen, A., Lee, C. W., Monson, C. M., … Bicanic, I. A. E. (2016). CRITICAL ANALYSIS OF THE CURRENT

TREATMENT GUIDELINES FOR COMPLEX PTSD IN ADULTS. *Depression and Anxiety*, *33*(5), 359–369. https://doi.org/10.1002/da.22469

Findings from the National Vietnam Veterans' Readjustment Study - PTSD: National Center for PTSD. http://www.ptsd.va.gov /professional/research-bio/research/vietnam-vets-study.asp

Herman, J. L. (1992). Complex PTSD: A syndrome in survivors of prolonged and repeated trauma. *Journal of Traumatic Stress*, *5*(3), 377–391. https://doi.org/10.1002 /jts.2490050305

Herman, J. L. (1997). *Trauma and Recovery*. Basic Books.

Herman, J. L., Perry, J. C., & van der Kolk, B. A. (1989). Childhood trauma in borderline personality disorder. *The American Journal of Psychiatry*, *146*(4), 490–495. https://doi .org/10.1176/ajp.146.4.490

Kolb, L. C., & Mutalipassi, L. R. (1982). The Conditioned Emotional Response: A Sub-Class of the Chronic and Delayed Post-Traumatic Stress Disorder. *Psychiatric Annals*, *12*(11), 979–987. https://doi.org /10.3928/0048-5713-19821101-06

Maercker, A., Brewin, C. R., Bryant, R. A., Cloitre, M., Reed, G. M., van Ommeren, M., …

Saxena, S. (2013). Proposals for mental disorders specifically associated with stress in the International Classification of Diseases-11. *Lancet (London, England)*, *381*(9878), 1683–1685. https://doi.org /10.1016/S0140-6736(12)62191-6

PTSD Becomes (More) Complex in the DSM-5: Part II | Psychology Today. https://www. psychology today.com/blog/hijacked-your-brain/ 201306/ptsd-becomes-more-complex-in-the-dsm-5-part-ii

PTSD in DSM-5: Understanding the Changes | Psychiatric Times. (2015, September 25). http://www.psychiatrictimes.com/ptsd/ptsd-dsm-5-understanding-changes

Resetting the Fear Switch in PTSD: A Novel Treatment Using Acoustical Neuromodulation to Modify Memory Reconsolidation. https:// www. aca-demia.edu/12532059 /Resetting _the_Fear_Switch_in_PTSD_A_Novel_Treat ment_Using_Acoustical_Neuromodulation_to _Modify_Memory_Reconsolidation

van der Kolk, B. ISTSS - ISTSS Online Learning Library. https://www.istss.org/ education-research /online-learning/ recordings.aspx? pid=AMREC11-04

van der Kolk, B. A. (1988). The trauma spectrum: The interaction of biological and social events in the genesis of the trauma response. *Journal*

of Traumatic Stress, *1*(3), 273–290.
https://doi.org/10.1002/jts. 2490010302

Wilson, J. P. (2014). *Trauma, Transformation, And Healing.: An Integrated Approach To Theory Research & Post Traumatic Therapy.* Routledge.

Wolf, E. J., Miller, M. W., Kilpatrick, D., Resnick, H. S., Badour, C. L., Marx, B. P., … Friedman, M. J. (2015). ICD-11 Complex PTSD in US National and Veteran Samples: Prevalence and Structural Associations with PTSD. *Clinical Psychological Science : A Journal of the Association for Psychological Science*, *3*(2), 215–229. https://doi. org/10. 1177/2167702614545480

Chapter Eight:

SLEEP DISORDER

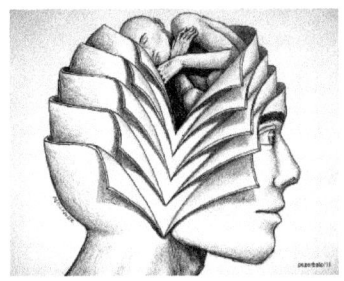

In the biblical tale of Job, God inflicts insomnia
on Job causing him to lament (Job 7:4), "When I lie
down, I say, 'When shall I rise, and the night be
gone?' And I am full of tossing to and fro
unto the dawning of the day."

"I've always envied people who sleep easily. Their
brains must be cleaner, the floorboards of the skull
well swept, all the little monsters closed up in a
steamer trunk at the foot of the bed."

David Benioff, City of Thieves

We begin this chapter with a section authored by my esteemed editor, Dr. James Miller, taken with his permission from his unpublished paper: *Fundamentals of Shift Work Scheduling, Third Edition: Fixing Stupid.* I provide this material as an overview of the cyclical stages of sleep as well as the effects that sleep deprivation has on normative functioning. The author notes that:

"Sleep is not a passive or vegetative state, as many assume. It is generated by complex activities in the brain. To emphasize this point, consider several complexities of sleep physiology. - Three kinds of sleep are identifiable with scalp electrodes (electroencephalogram, EEG).

"They are slow-wave sleep (SWS; sleep stages 3 and 4), rapid-eye-movement (REM) sleep, and stage 2 sleep. Generally, about half of a good-quality, normal night of sleep is spent in stage 2, while SWS and REM each occupy somewhat less than one-quarter of the night, and the remainder of the night is made up of drowsiness (stage 1) and wakefulness (stage 0) (Wolpert EA, 1969), (R. L. Williams, Karacan, & Hursch, 1974).

"The occurrence of SWS is associated with a release of growth hormone from the brain (Weibel, Follenius, Spiegel, Gronfier, & Brandenberger, 1997). Thus, we assume that SWS is a period during which some repair of muscle and nerve cells occurs, following their use during the preceding waking period(s). The occurrence of sleep is associated with memory consolidation ("System consolidation of memory during sleep,"). The proportions of sleep time spent in SWS and REM sleep depend quite a bit upon the degree and nature of sleep debt.

"The sleep stages mentioned above occur in an orderly manner with a 90-min cycle. When you first fall asleep in the evening and sleep through the night, you pass quickly through stages 1 and 2 into much-needed SWS. Eventually, you return to stage 2 and may generate some REM sleep. This cycle takes about 90 minutes. The cycle is repeated throughout the night with relatively less SWS and relatively more REM sleep as morning approaches.

"Five 90-minute cycles occur across 7½ hours. These five cycles plus some falling-asleep and waking-up times lead you to spend about eight hours in bed. . . Rough approximation of an eight-hour sleep histogram, showing the 90-minute cycle of sleep stages that occurs throughout the night.

"The brain regulates the amount of sleep that we need. This regulation operates somewhat like the thermostat on a furnace or air conditioner, generating a condition known as homeostasis: the ability or tendency of an organism or cell to maintain internal equilibrium by adjusting its physiological processes (American Heritage Dictionary). A thermostat triggers heating or cooling when the room temperature exceeds a defined range of temperature, driving the room temperature back toward a given "set point."

"Similarly, in the absence of sleep pathologies, when we are too sleepy, we are driven to fall asleep; and when we have recovered enough, we are driven to awaken. The need for sleep is a physiological drive, much like the drives for food and water.

"As with insufficient food and water intake, insufficient sleep leads to irritability and, if continued, to health problems. One may argue that sleep drive is even stronger than the drives to eat and drink. I may starve myself to death voluntarily or refuse to drink and then die of dehydration. However, continued sleep deprivation eventually causes each of us to fall asleep, initiating automatic recovery (Dr. James Miller)."

"No one gets used to not getting enough sleep. They might be able to do it, but they never overcome the drive for sleep or the consequences that invariably follow sleep restriction" (Caldwell & Caldwell, 2005). Sleep debt has been compared to borrowing from a bank." (Morgan, 1996)

"People who sleep less than 8 hours per 24 hours are taking "little 'loans' from their sleep banker." Morgan cautioned that "You know that your dangerously moody sleep banker may call in the loan when you are driving at 79 miles per hour on the freeway." You should "deposit eight hours in your sleep bank every day." In fact, the (about ages 25 to 70 years) is seven to nine hours per night." (Hirshkowitz et al., 2015)

"Sleep inertia occurs normally in the morning after awakening. It is a grogginess that usually lasts only about five minutes but may last up to 15 or 30 minutes in a person with a large, previous sleep debt. Though sleep inertia may not be detected as a problem after napping (Driskell & Mullen, 2005), it is possible that if the deeper stages of sleep occur during a nap, then this same sleep inertia may occur. Thus, at least 15 to 30 minutes should be allowed after a nap to allow sleep inertia to dissipate before performing safety-sensitive jobs.

"Humans have specific physiological and psychological requirements for getting adequate sleep. Everyone knows how it feels to get too little sleep. Sleepiness may be defined as an untimely desire to sleep and/or difficulty staying awake when wakefulness is required. Mental fatigue includes many symptoms, such as malaise, impairment of mood, memory impairment, slowed response time and impaired vigilance.

"Both sleepiness and mental fatigue are caused primarily by lack of sleep. When we do not get adequate sleep, we experience excessive mental fatigue during the time we are awake, also called excessive daytime sleepiness (EDS). EDS often affects our ability to perform our jobs safely. Repeated sleep loss of even one or two hours per night will eventually degrade alertness and mental performance significantly, with greater effects for greater amounts of sleep debt.

"The effects of one night of sleep deprivation, for example not sleeping for 40 continuous hours, can still be detected in performance levels after five nights of sleeping for six hours per night. (Jay et al., 2007)

"We measure both mood and mental performance during laboratory and field investigations of the effects of fatigue. Generally, fatigue-induced impairments of mood and of mental performance do not occur exactly in parallel. For example, after a night of sleep deprivation we may experience mood elevation when the sun comes up, but our mental performance may still be insidiously impaired

"Conversely, we may be convinced, again insidiously, that our mental performance is adequate even though we are feeling the malaise of fatigue. This latter situation leads to single-vehicle, run-off-the-road traffic accidents in which the driver falls asleep at the wheel. This latter situation also underscores the need to create fatigue-reduction strategies when we are well-rested, not when we are already fatigued. Fatigued people tend to make "stupid" decisions." (Mackie & Miller, 1978), (Woodrow, 2014)

Before proceeding, I'd like to share some information with you that can save you from developing cataract's early as well as from unnecessarily experiencing an altered sleep pattern in your own life. Since retiring from active practice and starting another career as an author and researcher, I spend a large amount of my time on the computer. Over the past two years, my sleep pattern has become increasingly erratic.

During my visit to Asheville, I scheduled an annual eye exam and discussed with my Optometrist, Dr. Larry Golson if there was any possible association between my sleep difficulties and my increased time on the computer. He informed that that there was definitely a linkage and it was due to the effects of 'blue light' emanating from the screen.

I was provided with new glasses that screen out the blue light and within one day, my sleep pattern began to normalize. No more naps needed during the day or waking up feeling unrested.

Please be aware of this if you spend much time looking at your screen and discuss it with your Optometrist. Blue light in the range of wavelengths 446–477 nm has been identified as the most potent light stimulus that suppresses melatonin production, a hormone that plays a major role in the regulation of sleep and wake cycles (Bossi & Hopker, 2016). Beyond obtaining protective lenses, there are computer programs such as flux that shut off the screen's blue emanations at night.

We now make a strategic shift from normative and sleep deprivation states to focus on disturbances in sleep, including nightmares as well as insomnia. Sleep disorders are all too common persevering symptoms that are present before and unfortunately after treatment for PTSD.

A 2016 study explored the prevalence of sleep difficulties in a sampling of active duty personnel with PTSD who had completed at least one deployment in Iraq or Afghanistan. The participants were randomly assigned to either a Group Cognitive Processing Therapy - Cognitive Only Version or assigned to a Group Present - Centered Therapy experience. Assessments were made prior to and following treatment for PTSD. The authors of the study concluded that:

> Insomnia was the most frequently reported symptom before and after treatment, with 92% reporting insomnia at baseline and 74%-80% reporting insomnia at follow-up. Nightmares were reported by 69% at baseline and by 49%-55% at follow-up. . . Insomnia was found to be one of the most prevalent and

persistent problems among service members receiving PTSD treatment. . . At baseline, 54% were taking sleep medications, but sleep medication use did not affect the overall results." (Ke et al., 2016).

The conceptualization of insomnia in the first half of the twentieth century was largely dominated by the psychoanalytic view of it as being a psychoneurotic symptom, treatable, in theory, through psycho-analysis. This view perpetuated the long-standing perception of insomnia as a symptom secondary to psychological distress for other primary conditions. Sateia, et. al., postulated that:

> The view of insomnia as a secondary symptom has largely persisted, even to the present day. However, as our understanding of the biological and psycho-behavioral character-istics of the condition has grown, greater emphasis has been placed on insomnia as a disorder in its own right, with a psycho-physiology that may be, in many respects, independent of the identified "primary" condition." (Sateia & Buysse, 2016)

I propose that the presence of continuing sleep disturbance with its accompanying symptoms described in the Ke et. al., article, represents a lack of change or alteration in the cortical brain circuitry that perpetuates the effects of PTSD. In fact, I would go so far as to postulate that continuance of sleep difficulties represent a failure of the treatment intervention to adequately alter the underlying neuronal structure. In my mind, this fact would become a primary yardstick for the measurement of success or failure of a specified PTSD treatment disorder.

An earlier study (2004) investigated whether insomnia continued following completion of a course of cognitive behavioral therapy (CBT). An analysis of scores from a 'gold standard' PTSD scale (CAPS) taken from 27 patients was used in the analysis. The participants were thought to be apparently free of PTSD symptoms at the completion of their treatment phase. Results of the study revealed that 48% of the participants continued to report residual insomnia. The researchers noted that:

> For the large majority, insomnia persisted in the absence of continuing nightmares and hypervigilance. Experiencing trauma in a sleep-related context was associated with greater risk for residual insomnia, whereas childhood abuse history and depression were not. These findings suggest that interventions to address factors maintaining insomnia residual to PTSD warrant study." (Zayfert & DeViva, 2004).

Unfortunately, while the most glaring symptoms of PTSD such as flashbacks and intrusive nightmares subside, our military personnel are left with residual aspects of the underlying condition over the remainder of their lives. I believe that the continuance of the symptom of insomnia alone is a contributing factor to late onset PTSD (LOPTSD) as well as early senescence findings in our aging combat involved Veteran population. (Lohr et al, 2015).

To state this in the form of a hypothesis, I would propose that unless all associated trauma symptoms such as sleep disturbance are absent, the neuronal circuitry that perpetuates PTSD remains activated. This is a 'red light,' 'green light' phenomena. To say it in a slightly different way, the 'fear switch' is either turned on or off – there is no dimmer switch in the system.

The framework for this chapter will constitute an exploration of sleep disturbance and its relationship to traumatic experiences. Some of the terms associated with the condition will be reviewed although a comprehensive discussion of the multiple forms of sleep disorder will not. This would best be left to those who specialize in the field.

Different characteristics of the condition will be explored such as nightmares and insomnia. I will also review the topic of breath obstruction and sleep apnea in the context of its relationship with trauma. Case examples will be interwoven throughout the chapter regarding dramatic changes in sleep patterns following the provision of RESET Therapy. These 'snippets' are taken from patients I have personally treated and written about in my first book: *PTSD Symptoms Reversed Permanently*. Please note my patient's comments as evidenced in their verbiage about the sleep related change that occurs when the 'trauma switch' turns off.

We begin the discussion with an exploration of prevalence rate in the older male Veteran population. Male Veterans ranging from age 55 to 89 volunteered for a study on post-traumatic stress disorder and cognitive decline. Questionnaires and overnight polysomnographic sleep studies were utilized. The researchers reported that:

"Undiagnosed sleep disordered breathing (SDB) was more than threefold higher than expected in these community-dwelling older veterans. . . Most were at high risk for sleep disorders including restless leg syndrome (53%), obstructive sleep apnea (66%), and circadian sleep disorders (72%). Forty-seven percent endorsed clinically significant symptoms of PTSD." (Mayer, Levy, Farrell-Carnahan, Nichols, & Raman, 2016)

****

(Shawn's therapist) Shawn underwent the neuromodulation procedure on our second visit and after about 15 minutes said his body 'felt loose'. To him, the traumatic event now seemed fuzzy when he tried to recall it. On a scale of 0 to 10, with 10 being the highest level of disturbance possible and 0 being no disturbance at all, he stated that his degree of disturbance had dropped from 10 to 1. The positive changes my client experienced during the week that followed included more normal sleep patterns, more tolerance for minor annoyances, less anger and more joy in life.

(Shawn) Looking back on it now, I know that the trauma changed me. I used to be compassionate and loving and I turned cold and callous. I used to be funny and people wanted to be around me and after, I wasn't funny like I used to be and I didn't like to be around people. After the trauma I noticed that I didn't sleep as much. I started having nightmares. I would see the burning bodies and I didn't want to see them anymore.

****

Let us now briefly explore what the term quality of sleep means:

Subjective sleep quality refers to perceived ease of falling asleep, staying asleep, and obtaining adequate sleep that leaves one feeling rested. Such perceptions do not necessarily correspond to objective measures of sleep quality provided by polysomnography. Nevertheless, they are the key to diagnosing some sleep disturbances, such as insomnia. (Newton & Fernandez-Botran, 2016)

The authors of the following article hold the belief that insomnia can be treated through Cognitive Behavioral Therapy - Insomnia Treatment that assists the patient to identify and change their beliefs system and accompanying behaviors that interfere with sleep. The study was conducted with 68 active duty United States military personnel (97% males) who had been deployed in the prior 18 months and diagnosed with insomnia. The authors noted that:

"Probable syndromal depression or post-traumatic stress disorder (PTSD) was present in 47 and 28% of participants, respectively. . . Participants were assessed before, and immediately after, completing treatment for insomnia (cognitive–behavioral therapy for insomnia) or for comorbid insomnia and obstructive sleep apnea (either sleep education or cognitive–behavioral therapy for insomnia combined with positive airway pressure). Assessments included subjective sleep quality, depression and posttraumatic stress symptoms, and peripheral blood gene expression profiles.

"After 3 months of treatment, two clusters of participants were identified, those with any improvement in subjective sleep quality (68% of the sample) and those without any improvement (32% of the sample)." (Koffel, Khawaja, & Germain, 2016)

There is no mention in the prior article of any of the subjects returning to a fully normative sleep pattern. It is not specifically clarified what level of improvement the patients obtained. It is clearly stated that 32% obtained no benefit from the treatment. I also find it interesting that the authors placed the majority group within a category described as: "those with any improvement in subjective sleep quality." That seems to me to be quite a wide group potentially ranging from minimal to major change in sleep status.

Another recent article (2016) reviewed the use of adjunctive risperidone in a "24-week multicenter randomized placebo-controlled trial of adjunctive risperidone in patients with chronic military-related PTSD symptoms (n = 267, 97% male) who were symptomatic despite treatment with antidepressants and other medications."

This study highlighted the near universality and significant negative impact of severe disturbances in sleep quality in veterans with chronic military-related PTSD who were partial responders to standard pharmaco-therapies. The modest improvements in sleep quality produced by adjunctive risperidone were correlated with limited reductions in PTSD severity and improvements in quality of life." (Krystal et al., 2016)

My review of a few recent studies that sought to address sleep disturbance in our combat Veterans revealed neither a therapeutic nor a pharmacologic approach that attained a level of success of total absence, both subjectively as well as objectively, of the symptoms of sleep disorder.

****

(Shawn) I would stay up late until I was totally exhausted and then pass out either on the couch or be woken up and told to go to bed. I figured   if I didn't dream, I wouldn't have the nightmares. On one occasion I actually hit my wife while I was asleep. While we were still together at Fort Bragg, North Carolina, I noticed the changes in myself and I couldn't figure it out.

I've seen the daily frustrated look erased from his face. Shawn's been able to deal with things and not go to that dark place he once knew. He has started to sleep better, has more patience and actually seems happy. I don't understand how the procedure worked but I know that it did. I got back that 'sweet Shawn' that I knew from high school." - Lynn

****

At this point in our discussion, let's clarify what nightmares are in the PTSD condition. The authors of the following article note that:

"Nightmares are a unique feature of posttraumatic stress disorder (PTSD). Although nightmares are a symptom of PTSD, they have been shown to independently contribute to psychiatric distress and poor outcomes, including heightened suicidality and suicide. Nightmares are often resistant to recommended pharmacological or psychological PTSD treatments." (Campbell & Germain, 2016)

Edition Three of the International Classification of Sleep Disorders (ICSD-3) has redefined nightmares as "repeated occurrences of extended, extremely dysphoric, and well-remembered dreams that usually involve threats to survival, security, or physical integrity" (Sateia, 2014). Nightmares are estimated to disturb the sleep of as many as 50 % of PTSD involved adults." (Regier et al., 2013)

A 2012 study that investigated nightmare characteristics and their association with treatment outcome found that PTSD combat Veterans' nightmares:

"were replete with scenes of death and violence and were predominantly replays of actual combat events in which the veteran was under attack and feared for his life. Although addressing or resolving the nightmare theme with rescripting was associated with a reduction in sleep disturbance, references to violence in the rescripted dream were related to poorer treatment outcome in nightmare frequency. . .

"The experience of olfactory sensations in nightmares, a possible index of nightmare intensity, was also related to poorer treatment response; . . . Imagery rehearsal for individuals with severe, chronic PTSD and fairly replicative nightmares may be most effective when the rescripted dream incorporates a resolution of the nightmare theme and excludes violent details. . .

"Reports of olfactory experiences during original nightmares predicted a smaller reduction in sleep disturbances, possibly due to the link between odor perception and emotional memory. Harb and colleagues reasoned that experiencing smells may indicate intensity of a nightmare because of the rudimentary nature of the brain systems responsible for olfactory processing." (Harb, Thompson, Ross, & Cook, 2012)

While this may clearly be feasible to accomplish within a practiced rescripted experience, I cannot conceive of how it will alter the actual dream experience itself. The 'white washed' version of the nightmare simply doesn't suffice. The primitive violent material comes from 'the fangs of the cobra' as I've discussed in my earlier books. The limbic system doesn't compromise; it must be fully and completely turned off from its constant state of hyper-arousal.

In a similar manner, the subject of intimacy often becomes problematic for those who have experienced trauma. A 2015 study utilizing 60 subjects split into two groups explored this aspect of functioning by comparing fears of intimacy between people with PTSD as contrasted to those members of a group of healthy controls. All of the participants were engaged in intimate relationships at the time of the study. The authors concluded that a:

"Higher prevalence of extreme sensory sensitivity, avoidance, and low registration was found among the study group. These patterns significantly correlated with impaired emotional responses associated with intimacy. Low registration and group membership predicted fears of intimacy." (Engel-Yeger, Palgy-Levin, & Lev-Wiesel, 2015)

To take the above perspective a step further, clinical reports by Vietnam Veterans complaining of intimacy difficulties following active duty has raised the question of an association between post-traumatic stress disorder (PTSD) and sexual dysfunction (SD). The authors of the following study specifically reviewed literature regarding sexual dysfunction in male veterans with PTSD. Their methodical search included the following data bases: PubMed, the Cochrane database, and PsycINFO with 123 results generated. The authors concluded that:

"All but one study found an increased and significant prevalence of SD among male veterans with PTSD, especially erectile dysfunction and decreased sexual desire. SD increased in patients with PTSD, with a prevalence between 8.4% and 88.6%; the large prevalence range were partly the result of methodological differences. . .

"Increasing evidence suggests a correlation between PTSD and SD, but still, relatively few studies have addressed these questions. Further investigation is needed into the correlation between PTSD and SD, preferably taking severity of PTSD symptoms into account, along with confounders such as use of psychotropic medication, somatic illness, drug and alcohol abuse, and comorbid psychiatric illness." (Bentsen, Giraldi, Kristensen, & Andersen, 2015)

A final reference to this topic is included. The authors of the following article postulate that that the topic of sexual dysfunction itself is frequently overlooked or avoided in the discussion between patient and doctor. It clearly appears to be a topic to be avoided in scientific research literature. Is this reminiscent of the Victorian era? At any rate, the aim of the authors of the article was to review the current literature regarding sexual dysfunction among male and female Veterans with PTSD. They found that:

"Sexual dysfunction, including erectile difficulties in males and vaginal pain in females, is common among Veterans with PTSD. Several underlying mechanisms may account for the overlap between PTSD and sexual dysfunction. Certain barriers may contribute to the reluctance of providers in addressing problems of sexual dysfunction in Veterans with PTSD.

"Conclusions: With the high likelihood of sexual dysfunction among Veterans with PTSD, it is important to consider the integration of treatment strategies. Efforts to further the research on this important topic are needed." (Tran, Dunckel, & Teng, 2015)

The following brief case study was contributed by Dr. Terry Zumwalt, Commander, Medical Corps, USNR, who served as an operating Obstetrician /Gynecological surgeon in a military hospital emergency room as well as in civilian outpatient gynecological surgery units. Dr. Zumwalt reported that:

"On any given day, upwards of 40% of my patients were sexually/physically abused with hyper-sympathetic stress reactions to pelvic examinations. A 60-year-old Navy RN who at twelve-years of age was sexually raped and strangled, requested assistance with this life-long disturbance which affected her ability to fully participate in intimacy with her significant other.

"I provided her with combined treatment consisting of MASER's (Military Grade Meridian Tapping) which is a variation of Emotional Freedom Therapy (EFT) and RESET Therapy. Consequently, her musculature, particularly in the genital region that was chronically tense, relaxed. After application of pressure and focus to the neck and shoulder region to address the strangulation aspect of her experience, her arms pushed away and her legs straightened. Her hands were shaking. The treatment stopped after she said she was 'done'.

"Two months later she called me to tell me that for 3-4 nights following the combined therapy session, her muscles repeated the shaking - pushing away moves as she was relaxing and going to sleep. As an aside, she reported that ever since the treatment, her orgasmic releases had become the most powerful ever. This occurred with just one RESET Therapy treatment during which she was able to image staring into the face of her attacker while listening to the binaural sound."

Another recent study provides us with a perspective of how persons who experience nightmares perceive of their condition. This includes their willingness to discuss details of their encounter with terror with a healthcare provider. Furthermore, they are asked if they perceive that their condition is treatable. The authors presented the following two-component conditions:

"In Study 1, participants (n = 809) were asked whether they had discussed nightmares with a healthcare provider. In Study 2, participants (n = 747) were asked whether they believed nightmares were treatable in addition to whether or not they had discussed nightmares with a healthcare provider.

"Of the participants in Study 1 experiencing clinically significant nightmare symptoms only 37.8% of participants reported discussing their nightmares with a healthcare professional. In Study 2, only 11.1% of participants with significant nightmares reporting having told a healthcare provider about their nightmares. Further, of these individuals with clinically significant nightmare symptoms, less than one-third believed that nightmares were treatable." (Nadorff, Nadorff, & Germain, 2015)

****

(Shawn) "I still don't really understand how this happened but with one treatment, my wife says I'm a changed man. I asked her what she meant and she said, when you came home from that treatment you've become that boy I fell in love with 25 years ago.

I can feel the change in me now. I laugh again. I enjoy life and I love my wife. Since my treatment, I had been able to sleep 8 hours a night like I used to with no flashbacks, no

nightmares and no survivor's remorse. Also,
since my treatment, I have lost 20 pounds,
have   more energy and I have come to enjoy life.

****

To finalize this discussion of nightmares, a 2013
study by Margolies et al. utilized a combined
cognitive-behavioral therapy for insomnia (CBT-I)
and imagery rehearsal therapy (IRT) for nightmares
to ascertain if these approaches were amenable
through these approaches. The following findings
were reported by the authors:

"The present study randomized 40 combat veterans
(mean age 37.7 years; 90% male and 60% African
American) who served in Afghanistan and/or Iraq
(Operation Enduring Freedom [OEF]/Operation Iraqi
Freedom [OIF]) to 4 sessions of CBT-I with
adjunctive IRT or a waitlist control group. Two thirds
of participants had nightmares at least once per week
and received the optional IRT module.

"At posttreatment, veterans who participated in CBT-
I/IRT reported improved subjectively and objectively
measured sleep, a reduction in PTSD symptom
severity and PTSD-related nighttime symptoms, and

a reduction in depression and distressed mood compared to the waitlist control group.

"The findings from this first controlled study with OEF/OIF veterans suggest that CBT-I combined with adjunctive IRT may hold promise for reducing both insomnia and PTSD symptoms. Given the fact that only half of the patients with nightmares fully implemented the brief IRT protocol, future studies should determine if this supplement adds differential efficacy to CBT-I alone." (Margolies, Rybarczyk, Vrana, Leszczyszyn, & Lynch, 2013)

■■

If I am interpreting the above findings correctly, no change in nightmares was forthcoming from the intervention. The authors speculated that this result may be due to differences in a military population or possible non-compliance of the study volunteers. Might the results have been due to the non-effectiveness of the treatment intervention itself?

✳✳✳✳✳✳✳✳✳✳✳✳✳✳✳✳✳✳✳✳✳✳✳✳✳✳✳✳

Joe decided to seek treatment with me stating that: "I've come to see you because I've been having bad dreams this past year and my wife has become afraid to touch me. If a car backfires, it kicks off panic reactions in me.

In his first RESET Therapy session, Joe reported that: "It all went away – It faded out. What happened is there but it didn't affect me that much. When we first started, my heart was going 90 miles a minute. My muscles were tense and tears started rolling. Then it wasn't there anymore. The emotions didn't come with it! I'm feeling at peace now.

****

Our next area of focus will be directed towards the topic of obstructive sleep apnea syndrome, obstructive sleep apnea syndrome (OSAS). As noted on WebMD:

"When you have this condition, your breath can become very shallow or you may even stop breathing -- briefly -- while you sleep. It can happen many times a night in some people. Obstructive sleep apnea happens when something partly or completely blocks your upper airway during shut-eye. That makes your diaphragm and chest muscles work harder to open the obstructed airway and pull air into the lungs. Breathing usually resumes with a loud gasp, snort, or body jerk. You may not sleep well, but you probably won't be aware that this is happening. The condition can also reduce the flow of oxygen to vital organs and cause irregular heart rhythms."

We'll begin this discourse with a 1998 report of a 42-yr-old man with PTSD and accompanying severe OSAS. I chose this study primarily due to the authors note that the patient's "PTSD symptoms abated when his OSAS was successfully treated." Thus, an early link between the two conditions in the literature was established before the turn of the century. The authors concluded that:

"This case supports the notion that treatment of PTSD will be more successful if treatment of sleep complaints is emphasized and if sleep apnea and other sleep disorders are treated aggressively. The possibility of a connection between sleep-disordered breathing and PTSD, as seen in this case, has implications for understanding the physiology and treatment of PTSD." (Youakim, Doghramji, & Schutte, 1998)

We will now leap to a 2015 study focusing on the relationship between obstructive sleep apnea (OSA) and psychiatric pathology. The authors state that: The goal of this study is to examine the prevalence and treatment of OSA in psychiatric populations.

"A systematic review . . . was conducted to determine the prevalence of OSA in schizophrenia and other psychotic disorders, mood disorders, and anxiety disorders, and to examine potential interventions. The PubMed, EMBASE, and PsycINFO databases were searched (last search April 26, 2014) using keywords based on the ICD-9-CM coding for OSA and the DSM-IV-TR diagnostic groups.

"Conclusions: OSA prevalence may be increased in MDD and PTSD. In individuals with OSA and psychiatric illness, treatment of both disorders should be considered for optimal treatment outcomes." (Gupta & Simpson, 2015)

****

Joe was skeptical that his results would be only temporary, so he asked if it would be alright to return for a number of follow-up sessions. He returned a week later reporting that he was sleeping better. "Previously, I was waking up every hour. I used to wake sitting straight up. I'm also remembering more things now that I previously couldn't think about."

During his second visit and 20 minutes of
RESET Therapy, Joe targeted all the newly
emerging memories that had surfaced into his
awareness. He reported that: "I went through
it   all and can't think of anything else. I'm
feeling   relaxed and could fall asleep right
now.

After his third treatment session, Joe's wife
reported: "He's doing better and not jumping
up and down every time I ask him to do
something. He sleeps better – no moaning. He
doesn't sit straight up in bed suddenly at
night. He has more patience with me now when we
shop." Joe added that, "We've been married
for 52 years, and she's been through it all. I
would give the world to her if I could.

****

At this point, we will focus on a younger group of
military personnel who have served in Iraq and
Afghanistan (OEF/OIF/OND) with self-reported
posttraumatic stress disorder (PTSD) symptoms and
the risk of obstructive sleep apnea (OSA). The
participants consisted of 195 Iraq and Afghanistan
veterans who presented for evaluation for PTSD at a

VA outpatient clinic. The following results were presented by the authors:

"Of 159 veterans screened, 69.2% were assessed as being at high risk for OSA. PTSD symptom severity increased the risk of screening positive for OSA. PTSD symptom severity increased risk of screening positive for snoring and fatigue, but not high blood pressure/BMI." (Colvonen et al., 2015)

In the next study, the focus was directed to active duty soldiers with deployment-related PTSD in order to assess the rate of sleep complaints and sleep disorders among them. The researchers recorded polysomno-graphic data as well as subjective measures of sleep. The researchers reported that:

"One hundred thirty patients were included (91.5 % male, mean age of 35.1 ± 10.6 years, . . . About 88.5 % had comorbid depression, with the majority (96.2 %) taking psychoactive medications . . . Over half of the cohort suffered combat-related traumatic physical injuries (54.6 %). The obstructive sleep apnea syndrome (OSAS) was diagnosed in 67.3 % (80 % of the cohort underwent polysomnography) . . . OSAS was significantly more common in the non-injured soldiers . . .

■■

"Sleep complaints are common among soldiers with PTSD. We observed significantly higher rates of OSAS among those without physical injuries, raising the possibility that underlying sleep-disordered breathing is a risk factor for the development of PTSD. This potential association requires further validation." (S. G. Williams, Collen, Orr, Holley, & Lettieri, 2015)

Let's look at another yet another example of RESET therapy with a veteran who was stuck in the chronic anger/fight stage of his PTSD condition. Robert served honorably in the Vietnam War as a gunner who was thrust headfirst into horrific experiences that are difficult for a human being to imagine. He has suffered for nearly 50 years from the after effects of this experience, unable to shake the traumatic memories that have haunted him.

He has struggled to cope with a sleep disorder, drug use and overwhelming anxiety further complicated by misdiagnosis, unsuccessful therapy, multiple hospital-izations, and numerous medications that left him numb and devoid of his personality. He is like tens of thousands of other vets who suffer in silence.

****

■■■

After I got back from Vietnam I had flashbacks and nightmares. For 15 to 20 years I was nothing but an alcoholic and a drug addict. I would bolt upright from sleep at night terrified because I thought I was in combat.

My flashbacks started a few months after returning. Some of the triggers were the smells of gunpowder, burning flesh or decomposition and fireworks.

****

Rapid eye movement sleep behavior disorder (RBD) is a parasomnia in which there is enactment, often violent, of dream mentation. Although this syndrome is frequently associated with neurologic disorders, psychiatric comorbidity is not typical. Husain et al., present a unique series of veterans with RBD. A high incidence of comorbidity with post-traumatic stress disorder is noted.

"In the study, the literature on RBD was reviewed, Furthermore, the coexistence of RBD and post-traumatic stress disorder was postulated. The authors suggest that it is possible that similar neuropathologic processes are responsible for both conditions, at times in the same patient (Husain, Miller, & Carwile, 2001)."

"In contrast to the older study, above, researchers in a 2015 study explored excessive motor activity in 93 patients during dreaming in association with loss of skeletal muscle tone. As described by the authors:

"The patients were seen at the Mayo Sleep Disorders Center between January 1, 1991 and July 31, 1995. Eighty-one patients (87%) were male. The mean age of RBD onset was 60.9 years (range 36-84 years) and the mean age at presentation was 64.4 years (37-85 years). Thirty-two per cent of patients had injured themselves and 64% had assaulted their spouses. . . Dream content was altered and involved defense of the sleeper against attack in 87%." (Wing, Lam, Tsoh, & Mok, 2015)

****

On his return visit one week later, Robert reported that, "I was thinking about the event and all but it seemed more peaceful. I haven't had any nightmares or flashbacks compared to previously having them 2 to 3 times per week." His wife reported that her husband had done some work on the car rather than just sitting despondently in the house.

Now he talks again and is carrying on conversations. He didn't do that before. He would just lay in bed with a dark look on his face eating and watching TV all the time. His communication is getting better and he is getting back to the way he used to be. He helps with the chores. The very first treatment he had was like a miracle. He went home, slept well, didn't jerk awake, didn't jump up awake slamming, screaming, looking like someone was going to kill him.

His wife noted that, "He hasn't been having any nightmares and doesn't jerk anymore at night. Overall he is improving."

****

The authors of the following 2015 journal article summarized their perspective pertaining to future research of the sleep underpinnings of PTSD. They state:

"Sleep research in PTSD samples (as well as in other stress-related disorders such as acute stress disorder, adjustment disorders, prolonged grief disorder) is ripe for the broader use of state-of-the-science sleep neuroimaging methods required to identify the sleep-specific neurobiological underpinnings of PTSD, the correlates of resistance to first-line PTSD treatments, the predictors of response to sleep-focused treatments, and the mechanisms that are normalized by effective sleep treatments.

"Understanding the sleep-specific mechanisms . . . may be especially important in samples where trauma exposure is a likely event, such as during military deployment, combat exposure, and all emergency responders. Further investigating the role of sleep in the consolidation of traumatic memories as well as in processing emotional and traumatic material also provides an ecologically valid paradigm to further expand cognitive neuroscience models of sleep and memory.

"In summary, the study of the neurobiological correlates of PTSD during sleep by using state-of-the-science sleep neuroimaging methods opens multiple opportunities to identify the sleep-specific underpinnings of this pervasive disorder, which in turn can inform the development of evidence-based interventions that normalize the underpinnings of

PTSD across the sleep-wake cycle." (Germain, Buysse, & Nofzinger, 2008)

SUMMARY

Sleep disorder appears to be an integral and core aspect of PTSD. The symptoms of insomnia and nightmare generally appear to be resistant to current available therapies. As noted in the Ke et al., study, "insomnia was the most frequently reported symptom before and after treatment, with 92% reporting insomnia at baseline and 74%-80% reporting insomnia at follow-up. Nightmares were reported by 69% at baseline and by 49%-55% at follow-up."

I find the above statistics to be abysmal with the provided treatments to be lacking in understanding of the underlying neuronal networks involved in the perpetuation of the symptoms. We learned in Chapter One that even when the symptoms are weakened or suppressed, they seemingly re-emerge in the form of delayed onset PTSD (DOPTSD) with the symptom of dementia added to the mix.

Based on the foundation of the reviewed literature; I have taken the position that continuance of sleep difficulties represents a failure of the treatment intervention to adequately alter the underlying neuronal structure. In a similar fashion, nightmares with accompanying olfactory sensations for those involved in combat has been seen as indicative of poor outcome to traditional treatments.

Avoidance of intimacy is yet another feature associated with the trauma experience that weakens not only the marital bond but also the very structure of the family system itself. An observation by Commander Zumwalt brings home the incidence of effect for those women with prior abuse. She reported that: "upwards of 40% of my patients were sexually/physically abused with hyper-sympathetic stress reactions to pelvic examinations." In her provided case example, the patient returned to normal and full responsivity with a combination of treatment including RESET Therapy

••

References

Caldwell, J. A., & Caldwell, J. L. (2005). Fatigue in military aviation: an overview of US military-approved pharmacological countermeasures. *Aviation, Space, and Environmental Medicine, 76*(7 Suppl), C39-51.

Campbell, R. L., & Germain, A. (2016). Nightmares and Posttraumatic Stress Disorder (PTSD).

Current Sleep Medicine Reports, 2(2), 74–80.
http://doi.org/10.1007/s40675-016-0037-0

Colvonen, P. J., Masino, T., Drummond, S. P. A.,
   Myers, U. S., Angkaw, A. C., & Norman, S.
   B. (2015). Obstructive Sleep Apnea and
   Posttraumatic Stress Disorder among
   OEF/OIF/OND Veterans. *Journal of Clinical
   Sleep Medicine: JCSM: Official Publication
   of the American Academy of Sleep Medicine,
   11*(5), 513–518. http://doi.org/10.5664/jcsm
   .4692

Driskell, J. E., & Mullen, B. (2005). The efficacy of
   naps as a fatigue countermeasure: a meta-
   analytic integration. *Human Factors, 47*(2),
   360–377.

Engel-Yeger, B., Palgy-Levin, D., & Lev-Wiesel, R.
   (2015). Predicting fears of intimacy among
   individuals with post-traumatic stress
   symptoms by their sensory profile. *The
   British Journal of Occupational Therapy,
   78*(1), 51–57. http://doi.org/10.1177/030
   8022614557628

Germain, A., Buysse, D. J., & Nofzinger, E. (2008).
   Sleep-specific Mechanisms Underlying
   Posttraumatic Stress Disorder: Integrative
   Review and Neurobiological Hypotheses.
   Sleep Medicine Reviews, 12(3), 185–195.
   http://doi.org/10.1016/j.smrv.2007.09.003

Gupta, M. A., & Simpson, F. C. (2015). Obstructive
   sleep apnea and psychiatric disorders: a

systematic review. *Journal of Clinical Sleep Medicine: JCSM: Official Publication of the American Academy of Sleep Medicine, 11*(2), 165–175. http://doi.org/10.5664/jcsm.4466

Harb, G. C., Thompson, R., Ross, R. J., & Cook, J. M. (2012). Combat-related PTSD nightmares and imagery rehearsal: nightmare characteristics and relation to treatment outcome. *Journal of Traumatic Stress, 25*(5), 511–518. http://doi.org/10.1002/jts.21748

Hirshkowitz, M., Whiton, K., Albert, S. M., Alessi, C., Bruni, O., DonCarlos, L., ... Adams Hillard, P. J. (2015). National Sleep Foundation's sleep time duration recommendations: methodology and results summary. *Sleep Health, 1*(1), 40–43. http://doi.org/10.1016/j.sleh.2014.12.010

Husain, A. M., Miller, P. P., & Carwile, S. T. (2001). Rem sleep behavior disorder: potential relationship to post-traumatic stress disorder. *Journal of Clinical Neurophysiology: Official Publication of the American Electroencephalographic Society, 18*(2), 148–157.

Jay, S. M., Lamond, N., Ferguson, S. A., Dorrian, J., Jones, C. B., & Dawson, D. (2007). The characteristics of recovery sleep when recovery opportunity is restricted. *Sleep, 30*(3), 353–360.

Ke, P., Dj, T., Js, W., J, M., S, Y.-M., Al, P., ... Pa, R. (2016). Residual Sleep Disturbances Following PTSD Treatment in Active Duty Military Personnel. *Psychological Trauma : Theory, Research, Practice and Policy*. Retrieved from http://europepmc.org/abstract/med/27243567

Koffel, E., Khawaja, I. S., & Germain, A. (2016). Sleep Disturbances in Posttraumatic Stress Disorder: Updated Review and Implications for Treatment. *Psychiatric Annals, 46*(3), 173–176. http://doi.org/10.3928/00485713-20160125-01

Krystal, J. H., Pietrzak, R. H., Rosenheck, R. A., Cramer, J. A., Vessicchio, J., Jones, K. M., ... Veterans Affairs Cooperative Study #504 Group. (2016). Sleep disturbance in chronic military-related PTSD: clinical impact and response to adjunctive risperidone in the Veterans Affairs cooperative study #504. *The Journal of Clinical Psychiatry, 77*(4), 483–491. http://doi.org/10.4088/JCP.14m09585

Mackie, R. R., & Miller, J. C. (1978). *Effects of Hours of Service Regularity of Schedules and Cargo Loading on Truck and Bus Driver Fatigue*. National Highway Traffic Safety Administration.

Margolies, S. O., Rybarczyk, B., Vrana, S. R., Leszczyszyn, D. J., & Lynch, J. (2013). Efficacy of a cognitive-behavioral treatment for insomnia and nightmares in Afghanistan and Iraq veterans with PTSD. *Journal of Clinical Psychology, 69*(10), 1026–1042. http://doi.org/10.1002/jclp.21970

Mayer, S. B., Levy, J. R., Farrell-Carnahan, L., Nichols, M. G., & Raman, S. (2016). Obese Veterans Enrolled in a Veterans Affairs Medical Center Outpatient Weight Loss Clinic Are Likely to Experience Disordered Sleep and Posttraumatic Stress. *Journal of Clinical Sleep Medicine: JCSM: Official Publication of the American Academy of Sleep Medicine, 12*(7), 997–1002. http://doi.org/10.5664/jcsm.5934

Morgan, D. (1996). *Sleep secrets for shift workers & people with off-beat schedules.* Whole Person Associates.

Nadorff, M. R., Nadorff, D. K., & Germain, A. (2015). Nightmares: Under-Reported, Undetected, and Therefore Untreated. *Journal of Clinical Sleep Medicine: JCSM: Official Publication of the American Academy of Sleep Medicine, 11*(7), 747–750. http://doi.org/10.5664/jcsm.4850

Newton, T. L., & Fernandez-Botran, R. (2016). Promoting Health by Improving Subjective Sleep Quality? Reduction in Depressive Symptoms and Inflammation as Potential Mechanisms and Implications for Trauma-

Exposed Persons. *Frontiers in Psychiatry*, *7*.
http://doi.org/10.3389/fpsyt.2016.00076

Regier, D. A., Narrow, W. E., Clarke, D. E.,
Kraemer, H. C., Kuramoto, S. J., Kuhl, E. A.,
& Kupfer, D. J. (2013). DSM-5 field trials in
the United States and Canada, Part II: test-
retest reliability of selected categorical
diagnoses. *The American Journal of
Psychiatry*, *170*(1), 59–70.
http://doi.org/10.1176/appi.ajp.2012.1207099
9

Sateia, M. J. (2014). International classification of
sleep disorders-third edition: highlights and
modifications. *Chest*, *146*(5), 1387–1394.
http://doi.org/10.1378/chest.14-0970

Sateia, M. J., & Buysse, D. (2016). *Insomnia:
Diagnosis and Treatment*. CRC Press.

System consolidation of memory during sleep. from
http:/www.ncbi.nlm.nih.gov/pmc/articles/PM
C3278619/

Tran, J. K., Dunckel, G., & Teng, E. J. (2015). Sexual
dysfunction in veterans with post-traumatic
stress disorder. *The Journal of Sexual
Medicine*, *12*(4), 847–855. http://doi
.org/10.1111/jsm.12823

Weibel, L., Follenius, M., Spiegel, K., Gronfier, C.,
& Brandenberger, G. (1997). Growth
hormone secretion in night workers.
Chronobiology International, *14*(1), 49–60.

Williams, R. L., Karacan, I., & Hursch, C. J. (1974). *Electroencephalography (EEG) of human sleep: clinical applications.* John Wiley & Sons.

Williams, S. G., Collen, J., Orr, N., Holley, A. B., & Lettieri, C. J. (2015). Sleep disorders in combat-related PTSD. *Sleep & Breathing = Schlaf & Atmung, 19*(1), 175–182. http://doi .org/10.1007/s11325-014-0984-y

Wing, Y. K., Lam, S. P., Tsoh, J. M. Y., & Mok, V. C. T. (2015). Rapid eye movement sleep behaviour disorder and psychiatry: a case-control study. *Hong Kong Medical Journal = Xianggang Yi Xue Za Zhi / Hong Kong Academy of Medicine, 21 Suppl 6,* 34–38.

Wolpert EA. (1969). A manual of standardized terminology, techniques and scoring system for sleep stages of human subjects. *Archives of General Psychiatry, 20*(2), 246–247. http://doi.org/10.1001/archpsyc.1969.017401 40118016

Woodrow, A. (2014). Cognitive Performance Research at Brooks Air Force Base, Texas, 1960-2009. *Aviation, Space, and Environ mental Medicine, 85*(4), 482–482.

Youakim, J. M., Doghramji, K., & Schutte, S. L. (1998). Posttraumatic stress disorder and obstructive sleep apnea syndrome. *Psycho somatics, 39*(2), 168–171. http://doi.or g/10.1016/S0033-3182(98)71365-9

Zayfert, C., & DeViva, J. C. (2004). Residual insomnia following cognitive behavioral therapy for PTSD. *Journal of Traumatic Stress, 17*(1), 69–73. http://doi.org/10.1023/B:JOTS.0000014679.31799.e7

Epilogue

The notion of strength and weakness, "suck it up and move on" permeates our concept of being a man. Because of the importance of this issue, I've decided to include some of Retired Army Colonel Miguel Howe's statement in this section of this book. The Col. noted on October 5, 2016 that:

"This week, there has been much conversation around veterans who "can't handle" the "horrors" of war, and experience "mental health problems." This character-ization reveals an all too common stigma of the invisible wounds of war. It is also wrong, reflects a broader lack of knowledge and misunderstanding around the injury and how to treat it, and has egregious consequences.

"Through my own military service and the work of the Bush Institute, I know scores of service members and veterans — men and women of all services, ranks, and skill sets — who have come home with invisible wounds. . .

"Some of the challenges with these injuries are not the injury itself, but the stigma associated with them. TBI and psychological health conditions like PTS are natural outcomes of war. With the proper care, the invisible wounds are treatable. But if the perception exists that by being injured, they are somehow weaker than their colleagues, warriors won't ask for help.

". . . Beyond stigma and misconceptions, barriers to accessing and receiving care prevent many of our warriors from connecting to the treatment that they need. Many treatment options exist for the invisible wounds of war; yet, studies have shown that less than half of military personnel and veterans who experience them actually receive any care due to individual, logistical, financial, systemic, and community barriers.

. . .All citizens have a duty to understand these issues, increase awareness, and build a system of care that empowers warriors to overcome their injuries – not just our leaders. Together, we can not only improve the health and well-being of these warriors, but continue to leverage their strength and leadership in the coming decades." (Howe, 2016)."

Assuming that you have read the prior eight chapters in this book, by this point I would think that you have seriously considered PTSD to indeed be a system disorder. It is a condition that affects both the body as well as the mind. You have also been introduced to two therapeutic interventions that each contribute to the remediation of the hidden wounds of war.

I consider these two interventions to be the 'peanut-butter sandwich' that can significantly alter both the emotional as well as cognitive damage created by war incurred injuries. While my focus has been on combat Veterans, this same combination offers significant opportunity to civilians damaged through varied traumas as well as physically incurred injuries.

The first treatment (peanut-butter), of course is RESET Therapy as applied to PTSD as well as seven other conditions where the neuro-acoustical, binaural sound was described. The second component (jelly) as detailed in Chapter Two, harnesses the power of red-infra-red light. The bread in the sandwich is the skilled, trained and certified therapist guiding the patient through the remediative process.

Rather than providing you with a review of each chapter, I prefer to highlight stand-out aspects. Researching material for the book was certainly an eye-opening experience for me. For example, in Chapter One, you were introduced to startling information concerning the delayed onset (DOPTSD) of PTSD and the likely consequences forthcoming for our aging Veteran population.

In the following chapter, you were introduced to the world of "healing light" beginning with a detailed case study of Sergeant David Emme's experience with bTBI. Might red-infra-red light be the break-through non-invasive means for remediating not only TBI but also, dementing disorders as well?

Chapter Three featured pain sensitized circuits that become locked in a hyperactive state. I speculated that up to 80-90% of chronic pain can be eliminated through the use of binaural sound. What an impact this could make in regards to overuse and abuse of medication used for pain management.

In the following chapter, we focused on the seminal topic of depression. A number of studies revealed co-occurrence rates of around 50% among those with PTSD. RESET-Depression targeted to alter circuitry in the Lateral Habenula (LHb) was described in detail.

In Chapter Five, the focus was survivor's guilt and moral injury. As a clinician treating this condition, I have challenged whether 'Survivor's Guilt' is a distinct and separate disorder in its own right.

I have issues with the suggested six-month wait period when it is proposed that the condition changes from that of a normal grieving process to that of a pathological grief process. I also proposed that group therapy is not initially a treatment of choice for those who remain frozen in the protective/defensive mode created through the onset of trauma.

The topic of addiction was the focus in the following chapter. I proposed that trauma is frequently at the core of the addictive personality. Note was made that 40% of U.S. military veterans have a lifetime history of alcohol use disorder (AUD). Clearly, we must find treatments that can rapidly alter the cortical circuitry that sustains the addictive process. Chapter Seven addressed the topic of Complex PTSD with a detailed case study provided that exemplifies the treatment process.

Finally, the last chapter addresses the topic of sleep disorder. Based on my research and treatment provided in this area, I have concluded that unless insomnia and flash-backs/nightmares are totally and completely eliminated, the purported treatment has failed in fully remediating the total systemic effects that PTSD has on the spirit, body and mind.

In concluding, I invite you to continue this journey with me as I venture into my next book focused on the 'First Responders' among us. These heroes who serve us in our communities also pay the price for the trauma they must encounter. I look forward to sharing the application of RESET Therapy to this 'at-risk' population.